The
PCOS
Protection Plan

The
PCOS
Protection Plan

How to cut your increased risk of diabetes,
heart disease, high blood pressure and obesity

Colette Harris
Theresa Cheung

HAY HOUSE
Australia • Canada • Hong Kong
South Africa • United Kingdom • United States

First published and distributed in the United Kingdom by Hay House UK Ltd,
Unit 62, Canalot Studios, 222 Kensal Rd, London W10 5BN. Tel.: (44) 20 8962 1230;
Fax: (44) 20 8962 1239. www.hayhouse.co.uk

Published and distributed in the United States of America by Hay House, Inc.,
PO Box 5100, Carlsbad, CA 92018-5100. Tel.: (760) 431 7695 or (800) 654 5126;
Fax: (760) 431 6948 or (800) 650 5115. www.hayhouse.com

Published and distributed in Australia by Hay House Australia Ltd,
18/36 Ralph St, Alexandria NSW 2015. Tel.: (61) 2 9669 4299; Fax: (61) 2 9669 4144.
www.hayhouse.com.au

Published and distributed in the Republic of South Africa by Hay House SA (Pty), Ltd,
PO Box 990, Witkoppen 2068. Tel./Fax: (27) 11-706 6612. orders@psdprom.co.za

Distributed in Canada by Raincoast, 9050 Shaughnessy St, Vancouver, BC V6P 6E5.
Tel.: (604) 323 7100; Fax: (604) 323 2600

None of this book is intended to take the place of appropriate medical care. Please seek
professional help with any medical concerns you may have and do not attempt to treat or
diagnose symptoms in yourself or others (including animals) without taking professional
medical advice.

A catalogue record for this book is available from the British Library.

ISBN 1-4019-0539-0

Typeset by Scribe Design Ltd, Ashford, Kent, UK

Printed in Great Britain by TJ International, Padstow, Cornwall

Contents

Part Three: Success

Part Four: PCOS-Friendly Recipes   263

Preface

Are you, or someone you know, experiencing unexplained weight gain, irregular or non-existent periods, acne, thinning hair or unwanted facial hair growth? If you are, the chances are fairly good that you, or they, have polycystic ovary syndrome (PCOS).

Having PCOS is no fun. We know - we have PCOS ourselves, and it can make supposedly simple things seem complicated.

Perhaps you find it hard to lose weight however hard you try. Perhaps you've no idea when, or if, you'll get your next period. Perhaps you spend hours every morning and evening plucking and shaving unwanted and embarrassing facial and body hair. Perhaps the quality of your day is determined by whether or not your acne flares up. Perhaps thinning hair makes you feel older than you are, or perhaps tender swollen breasts, mood swings and endless fatigue make each day feel like an uphill struggle. Or perhaps you don't have many symptoms, or the ones you have you've learned to cope with.

But what about those other hidden problems that come with PCOS? The ones you don't see every day? These are the long-term complications such as an increased risk of diabetes, high blood pressure, heart disease and obesity.[1] That's why this book is called *The PCOS Protection Plan* – because using the advice in it helps you cut your risk of those life-threatening conditions that can accompany PCOS.

Today, it's estimated that as many as one in ten women has PCOS,[2] and even young girls are being diagnosed with the condition. Because this means that many sufferers will live with the condition for decades to come, their probability of developing complications is high. But equally, it means that they – and we – have a chance to take action sooner than ever before to cut the risk of these complications right back.

Rather than risking a bleak future, it's much better to take steps *now* that will reduce the chances that you'll ever develop complications. It may mean making some effort to live a healthier lifestyle, but if you can make that effort today you can avoid having to make a ton of effort and sacrifice tomorrow. And best of all, the basic diet and lifestyle changes recommended in this book will help you feel better *now*, as well.

If we'd known 10 years ago what we know now about PCOS, we could have avoided years of frustration and poor health. Since the time when we were both diagnosed – in the early to mid-nineties – we've learned a lot about this condition and how to manage it successfully. We've written books and articles about PCOS, spoken at conferences and support groups, and want to continue sharing all the information and research we've gathered about improving health and well-being if you've got PCOS. We've seen how PCOS symptoms, like acne, facial hair or hair loss can be early warning signs of serious problems that shouldn't be ignored.

We hope that *The PCOS Protection Plan* will inform you, prepare you and inspire you to take control of your health and prevent the serious complications associated with PCOS. And most of all, we hope it will inspire you to share your successes and ideas with other women, to help them cope, too.

Colette Harris
Theresa Cheung

1. Buccola, J. M. *et al.*, 'Polycystic ovary syndrome: a review for primary providers', *Prim Care* 2003 Dec; 30 (4): 697–710
2. Carmina, E. *et al.*, 'Diagnosis of polycystic ovary syndrome: from NIH criteria to ESHRE-ASRM guidelines', *Minerva Ginecol* 2004 Feb; 56 (1): 1–6

Acknowledgements

I'd like to thank Theresa, for her unfailing enthusiasm and great ideas in writing this book; Hay House for their support and professionalism; the experts and scientists researching PCOS for helping to inform us all; the women who have talked to us and inspired us with their questions and desire to take control of their health; the girls at Verity for doing such a good job; my friends and family for their understanding of my own PCOS; and finally, my father Chris for his constant care and encouragement of me in tackling this condition.

Colette

I'd like to thank Colette, for being such a joy to work with; Hay House for their help and support and attention to detail; the women with PCOS who shared their stories with us; and all the experts who gave us their time and shared their research with us. Last but by no means least, I'd like to thank Ray for his love and encouragement and my two lovely children, Robert and Ruth, for their love and patience.

Theresa

Introduction

WHAT IS PCOS?

Before you can get to grips with what you can do to reduce your risks of getting the serious problems associated with PCOS, you need to be clear about what PCOS is, what causes it, and which risk factors you can and can't change.

Basically PCOS, or polycystic ovary syndrome, is a complex hormonal and metabolic imbalance that affects your entire body and has lots of different effects on your health and well-being. Signs and symptoms include irregular or absent periods, infertility, insulin resistance, high cholesterol, unwanted facial body hair, thinning hair, acne and unexplained weight gain.[1]

WHAT CAUSES IT?

For many years PCOS was thought to be a direct result of high levels of male hormones – androgen (testosterone and so on)[2] – in the body, although no one seemed to know what caused these high levels. But researchers are now beginning to understand the link between PCOS, high androgen levels and an overproduction of insulin.[3] Insulin is a hormone that is normally released from the pancreas after a meal. It allows the cells of your body to take up energy from sugar, in the form of glucose. Glucose is also stored as *glycogen* by the liver.

It's crucial that your blood sugar (glucose) is maintained at a stable level, because brain function and the way your food is broken down and used for energy (metabolism) depend on it. When glucose levels are not properly controlled, diabetes is the inevitable result. If levels are too high (hyperglycaemia) this can cause excessive thirst, frequent urination and fainting. If levels are too low (hypoglycaemia) this can cause dizziness, headaches, shakiness and confusion. If you eat too much glucose than can be stored by the liver as glycogen, the excess is stored into fat cells and the result is weight gain.

INSULIN RESISTANCE

Studies have shown that many women with PCOS are insulin resistant.[4] This means the cells in your body aren't as sensitive to insulin as they would be normally, so you have problems converting glucose to energy. In an effort to compensate, your pancreas produces more insulin to try and get your cells to respond, so you end up with higher levels of circulating insulin than normal – a condition called hyperinsulinemia.

This excess insulin has a knock-on effect throughout your endocrine system, creating an imbalance with other hormones by stimulating higher-than-normal levels of male hormones which cause many PCOS-related symptoms such as irregular periods, acne and unwanted hair growth. Although not all women with PCOS are insulin resistant, many are, especially those with weight problems, because when weight goes up insulin levels tend to increase, too. If it's left untreated, insulin resistance can lead to weight gain and diabetes.

Insulin resistance, also known as Syndrome X, is a growing problem in the West where we eat a diet high in sugar and carbohydrates – the main cause of the condition.

A FAMILIAL LINK

Many leading researchers believe that PCOS has a hereditary component.[5] As Dr James Douglas – PCOS expert and reproductive endo-

crinologist at the Plano Medical Center in Texas – says, 'A familial dispo-
sition to the condition is very common.' In other words, if your mother
had irregular periods and (possibly undiagnosed) PCOS, it's likely that
you'll have it, too. So you need to do a little research and see if there's
a family history of diabetes, infertility, hirsutism (excessive hair growth)
and/or obesity. In the same way, inherited obesity can also increase your
risk of developing PCOS, because the more overweight you are the
worse your symptoms are likely to be, as fatty tissues produce excess
oestrogen, which can contribute to the overall hormone imbalance.

A brief history of PCOS

PCOS has mystified researchers for almost a century, since it was first
defined in 1935 by American gynaecologists Dr Irving Stein and Dr Michael
Leventhal. They were the first to link the seemingly unrelated symptoms –
lack of periods, abnormal hair growth, obesity and ovary enlargement due
to cysts – and give it a name. Later, the disorder was called polycystic ovary
syndrome because of the multiple 'cysts' found on the ovaries of many of
the women affected.

There's some debate today on the appropriateness of the name PCOS, as
not all women have the same symptoms. In PCOS, the 'cysts' are in fact
empty egg follicles that are just waiting for the right hormonal signal so
they can work properly; they are not the same as the large single cysts
that can develop and are simply known as ovarian cysts. 'So "polycystic" is
something of a misnomer,' says PCOS and ovary expert Helen Mason,
Senior Lecturer in Reproductive Endocrinology at St George's Medical
School, London. 'Many of us wish it had been called polyfollicular ovary
syndrome, but we are rather stuck with the name now.'

Alternative names that have been used or suggested include Syndrome O,
cystic ovaries, functional hyper-androgenism, Stein-Leventhal syndrome,
chronic anovulation and ovarian dysmetabolic syndrome. There are signs
that women with PCOS and the doctors who treat them are beginning to
see the need for a more consistent name that can better describe the
condition and prevent confusion in diagnosis and treatment, but for now
the term PCOS is here to stay.

Some studies suggest that women with PCOS may be born with a faulty gene that triggers higher-than-normal levels of androgen or insulin.[6] Researchers are now certain that the two biochemical markers of PCOS – high levels of insulin and testosterone – are linked. A study published in the US journal *Proceedings of the National Academy of Sciences* has suggested this link is a gene called follistatin which has two tell-tale functions: it plays a role in the development of the ovaries and is needed to make insulin.[7] Research into the genetics of PCOS continues.

Some experts believe that stress may be a contributory factor, so stress-reduction techniques are often recommended for women with PCOS.[8] More research is being done into this link, but in a way it's simply common sense: we all know that worry and anxiety can make your periods late, so it follows that stress can affect your hormones and therefore your PCOS symptoms in the same way.

Syndrome O

Syndrome O is the term some experts are using to describe the combination of two factors: insulin resistance and problems with ovulation in women. These basic problems lead to an array of women's health issues – abnormal bleeding, missed periods, infertility, acne, unwanted hair growth and high-risk pregnancies.

To be diagnosed with Syndrome O, both insulin resistance and problems with ovulation would need to be present. A diagnosis of PCOS, however, does not necessarily include insulin resistance. It's also worth pointing out that some women with PCOS symptoms don't actually have significant 'cysts' or empty follicles when checked with ultrasound.

Syndrome O – with its focus on insulin resistance in relation to problems with ovulation – does highlight something very important about the symptoms associated with PCOS. Since the majority of women with PCOS are insulin resistant, it's important to remind ourselves that the symptoms are not just caused by ovarian and sex hormone imbalances – they are also caused by metabolic disturbance and the long-term health risks this can trigger.

IS PCOS CURABLE?

PCOS is a bodily malfunction for which there's no cure, but if you have it you shouldn't tell yourself that you've got an incurable disease. You can't change the fact that you may be susceptible to PCOS, but you can make sure that your symptoms don't destroy the quality of your life. 'Diet and lifestyle changes,' says PCOS expert Dr Adam Balen, Professor of Reproductive Medicine and Surgery at Leeds General Infirmary in the UK, 'are without doubt your best defence. Your symptoms can be controlled with diet and lifestyle changes either by themselves or in combination with medical treatments and, perhaps, complementary therapies.'

Many women find that with the right diet and lifestyle changes, symptoms disappear. If you find the prospect of change daunting, remind yourself that if this means improved health and well-being and a better quality of life, not just now but in the future, it's well worth the effort.

'The biochemistry of PCOS is fascinating,' says Dr Adam Carey, PCOS expert, endocrinologist and co-founder of the London Nutrition Centre, 'but even more gripping is the realization that here is a genetic condition where, although there's no cure, sufferers can control the outcome through diet and lifestyle. It's a condition where women really can use their environment to interact with their genetic programming and create a positive outcome.'

Dr Carey acknowledges that the importance of diagnosing PCOS early, so a woman has time to make the appropriate lifestyle changes, is only just beginning to filter down from hospital consultants to doctors and GPs. 'There's still a long way to go, but it helps that the condition is starting to move out of the corridors of gynaecology and seen as a metabolic condition with a genetic basis in its own right. The idea that it's one of the first conditions to give sufferers the power to affect the expression of their own genes – a kind of natural genetic engineering – will make it a part of the biggest sea change in the practice of medicine in the first decade of 21st-century medicine.'

A BLESSING IN DISGUISE?

66 *This sounds odd but being diagnosed with PCOS was the best thing to have happened to me. Before I was diagnosed, my eating was out of control and I didn't exercise. I was a good 3 stone overweight. When the doctor told me I had PCOS and an increased risk of heart disease, obesity, diabetes and infertility, it was the wake-up call I needed. I was eating myself into an early grave. I ditched the unhealthy lifestyle. I asked my doctor for some diet and exercise guidelines, and within eight months my symptoms eased and I lost over 4 stone (56 lb). Everyone keeps asking me what my secret is — I tell them that it's the motivation PCOS gives me to take charge of my health and reduce the risk of life-threatening illness.* 99

Sonia, 36

Strange as it may seem, PCOS does have its positives. It can act as an early warning system to alert you that you're on the road to fertility problems, diabetes, heart disease, high blood pressure, obesity and all their associated complications, giving you the chance to do something about them before they strike.

HOW CAN THIS BOOK HELP?

This book offers a protective action plan to help you reduce your PCOS-associated health risks for the long term by taking steps with your diet, lifestyle and healthcare. As well as helping prevent future threats to your health, our action plan is also carefully designed to help reduce day-to-day symptoms such as acne, unwanted hair growth, hair loss, irregular periods, infertility, insulin resistance and weight gain. Our aim is to inspire you to enhance your overall health and vitality, both now and in the future. You can't lose!

But before you take action, you need to know why PCOS puts you at risk, and hear the evidence. That's why Part One of this book takes a look at the proven long-term health risks of PCOS.

REFERENCES

1. Aherne, S.A. *et al.*, 'Polycystic ovary syndrome', *Nurs Stand* 2004 Mar 10–16; 18 (26): 40–4

2. Azizz, R. *et al.*, 'Androgen excess in women: experience with over 1000 consecutive patients', *J Clin Endocrinol Metab* 2004 Feb; 89 (2): 453–62

3. Schroder, A. K. *et al.*, 'Insulin resistance in polycystic ovary syndrome', *Wien Klin Wochenschr* 2003 Dec 15; 115 (23): 812–21

4. Bernard, L. *et al.*, 'Insulin resistance and polycystic ovary syndrome', *Gynecol Obstet Fertil* 2003 Feb; 31 (2): 109–16

5. Atimo, W. H. *et al.*, 'Familial associations in women with polycystic ovary syndrome', *Fertil Steril* 2003 Jul; 80 (1): 143–5; Gonzalez, C. A. *et al.*, 'Polycystic ovaries in childhood: a common finding in daughters of PCOS patients. A pilot study', *Hum Reprod* 2002 Mar; 17 (3): 771–6

6. Strauss, J. F. *et al.*, 'Some new thoughts on the pathophysiology and genetics of polycystic ovary syndrome', *Ann N Y Acad Sci* 2003 Nov; 997: 42–8; Carey, A. *et al.*, 'Evidence for a single gene effect causing polycystic ovaries and male pattern baldness', *Clin Endocrinol (Oxf)* 1993 Jun; 38 (6): 653–8

7. Urbanek, M. *et al.*, 'Thirty seven candidate genes for PCOS: Strongest evidence of linkage is follistatin', *Proc Natl Acad Sci* 1999 July 20; 96 (15): 8573–8

8. Marantides, D. *et al.*, 'Management of polycystic ovary syndrome', *Nurse Pract* 1997 Dec; 22 (12): 34–8, 40–1

Part One
The Health Risks
Associated with PCOS

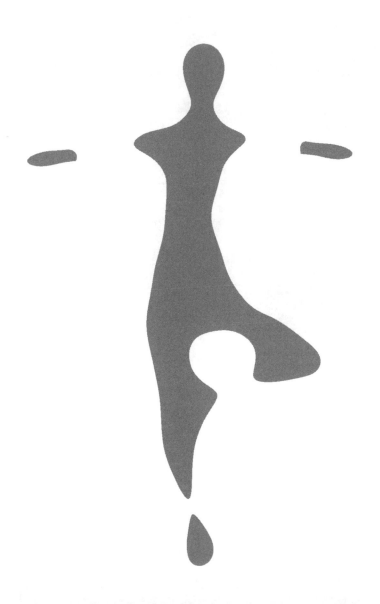

Introduction

Since the late 1990s, when women with PCOS finally began to get due attention from their doctors and the medical profession, the main issues under focus have been the day-to-day symptoms, from acne, facial hair and hair loss to depression and fertility issues – the things that can make living with PCOS seem such a frustrating struggle in the here and now.

Now that PCOS is on the map, and more research is being carried out than ever before to try and explain it, we've realized that for many women with PCOS, it's not just about coping with day-to-day symptoms; they're potential ticking time-bombs of serious health complications. Women like us with PCOS have an increased risk of diabetes,[1] heart disease,[2] high blood pressure,[3] obesity[4] and its related risks, and certain hormonal cancers.[5] It's time we and the medical professionals who support us really get to grips with reducing our risks for the future as well as our symptoms right now.

But exactly how great are these risks? And how is PCOS linked to conditions like heart disease and hormonal cancers? We'll look, risk by risk, at the links between PCOS and long-term health problems, giving you a chance to hear what the experts say about the risks and what you can do about them.

1. Pelusi, B. *et al.*, 'Type 2 diabetes and the polycystic ovary syndrome', *Minerva Ginecol* 2004 Feb; 56 (1): 41–51
2. Talbott, E. O. *et al.*, 'Cardiovascular risk in women with polycystic ovary syndrome', *Obstet Gynecol Clin North Am* 2001 Mar; 28 (1): 111–33
3. Rajkhowa, M. *et al.*, 'Polycystic ovary syndrome: a risk for cardiovascular disease', *BJOG: Int J Obstet Gynecol* 107 (1) Jan 2000: 11–18
4. Gonzalez, C. A. *et al.*, 'Polycystic ovarian disease: clinical and biochemical expression', *Ginecol Obstet Mex* 2003 May; 71: 253–8
5. Radulovic, A. *et al.*, 'Obesity and hormone function changes in female patients with polycystic ovaries', *Med Pregl* 2003 Sep-Oct; 56 (9–10): 476–80

1 Diabetes and Insulin Resistance

'I'm sorry, but you have diabetes.'

These words are heard by an estimated 18 million Americans and 2 million Britons every year. Not only will each person be affected but also the people close to them as well. Diabetes isn't just troubling, it can be dangerous: it's currently one of the top ten leading causes of death in the UK and the US.

Basically, diabetes means the level of sugar in your blood is too high. When we say sugar we don't mean table sugar (sucrose) but glucose, sometimes simply referred to as blood sugar. We all have glucose in our blood – we need it to provide energy to our cells – but when you've got diabetes you've got too much of a good thing. Having too much glucose in your blood can have serious consequences, increasing the risk of blockages in the arteries, which increase your risk of heart disease, stroke and kidney failure. Damage to small blood vessels in the feet can cause gangrene of the toes, while damage to the tissues at the back of the eye may cause loss of vision.

Blood sugar levels are high in people with diabetes because they have a problem with insulin. Insulin is the hormone that helps glucose get into your cells to be burned for energy. When insulin isn't doing its job, glucose can't get into your cells and accumulates in your blood, so that blood sugar levels just get higher and higher.

WHAT CAUSES DIABETES?

There are two main types of diabetes, and each type is caused by different things.

Type I diabetes, which usually begins in childhood or adolescence, can be genetic or brought on later by infections or viruses that damage the pancreas, or damage to the pancreas caused by chronic alcohol consumption. People with Type I diabetes don't produce enough insulin and need to inject insulin to bring their blood sugar levels down.

Type II diabetes usually occurs later in life and is the most common form of diabetes, making up to 95 per cent of all cases that occur in adults. People with Type II diabetes usually produce plenty of insulin but they have insulin resistance, which means that for some reason – and medical experts are still unsure of precisely why – their insulin doesn't work very well. People with Type II diabetes can reduce their insulin resistance and bring their blood sugar glucose levels down with diet and lifestyle changes and sometimes with drugs and insulin injections as well.

It's Type II diabetes that women with PCOS have a sevenfold increased risk of developing, so let's look at it in more detail.

While some studies suggest a genetic link, there's no 100 per cent certainty you'll develop diabetes even if a close family member has it. Clearly there are lifestyle factors at work – good news, because these are the things we do have control over.

People with Type II diabetes are often overweight and eat a poor diet. These factors have led many doctors and researchers to believe that an unhealthy lifestyle can contribute to the development of diabetes. A good example of this is the Pacific Islanders of Nauru, who became very wealthy when phosphates (used in detergents) were discovered on their island. As a consequence their lifestyle and eating habits changed dramatically and they put on a lot of weight and became more prone to developing diabetes.

Other studies suggest that the onset of diabetes can be related to a stressful event such as an accident or illness. All of this points to important connections between diet, environment, lifestyle and diabetes – invaluable information if you have PCOS.

WHAT'S MY RISK?

66 *Being diagnosed with PCOS when I was 19 was depressing enough; then two years later to be diagnosed with diabetes as well was a nightmare. My life's been turned upside down.* **99**

Kim, 24

66 *I've got PCOS and I'm a diabetic. At first I thought I must just be extremely unlucky to have both conditions, but when I joined PCOSA and started contributing to the message boards, the chat and got an e-mail buddy list, I soon realized that I wasn't alone — loads of women with PCOS have diabetes.* **99**

Gillian, 29

PCOS is a risk factor for diabetes[1] and if you've got PCOS you're up to seven[2] times more likely to get this condition. Research shows that if you're also insulin resistant and have problems managing your weight, you're perhaps the most vulnerable.[3] Some studies also suggest that women with irregular or absent periods may have double the risk for diabetes, and this risk increases again if irregular periods are paired with insulin resistance and/or obesity.[4]

It's estimated that at least half of all women with PCOS have insulin resistance. Insulin resistance has been linked to the development of diabetes, so if you've got PCOS and are insulin resistant, it's clear that you're at serious risk of developing diabetes at some point in your life.[5] In fact, everyone who develops Type II diabetes most likely has insulin resistance first, and because the connection is so strong many experts call insulin resistance 'pre-diabetes'.

The problems caused by insulin resistance (pre diabetes) just get worse until the body is no longer able to utilize insulin at all. The result is full-blown diabetes.

How can you tell when insulin resistance becomes diabetes? You need to ask your doctor to check your insulin levels or for a urine test to measure sugar levels.

When Does Insulin Resistance Become Diabetes?

The major portion of any meal you eat gets turned into glucose for your body to use. Insulin is the hormone that helps your body to access the sugar in your blood to use for energy. If you're insulin resistant (and many women with PCOS are), it means that your insulin doesn't work very well and so you can't efficiently burn the food you eat, even though your body will pump out higher-than-normal amounts of insulin to try and correct the situation. This means you have more insulin circulating in your body than normal, and that, while your body can still control the amount of sugar in your blood, it has to work twice as hard to do so.

Diabetes takes this a stage further: you have very poor control over the sugar in your blood, full stop.

So how does one turn into the other? After many years of producing greatly increased amounts of insulin, the insulin-producing cells in the pancreas start to wear out and stop working. Insulin levels then fall, blood sugar levels rise and rise, and full-blown diabetes sets in.

Insulin resistance would be diagnosed if your fasting insulin level (that is, the level after you've not eaten for 12 hours or more) is higher than 10 mlU/ml.[6] Another method is a glucose tolerance test (GTT), which shows how blood sugar levels change after a sugary drink, and checking insulin along with blood sugar levels. If the insulin level two hours after you have had a sugary drink is five times your fasting level, insulin resistance is diagnosed.

Other terms you might hear that indicate yet another step closer toward diabetes are *hyperinsulinaemia* (when insulin levels are high in relation to glucose levels), *impaired fasting glucose* (when the fasting glucose level is greater than 110 but less than 126 mg/dl) and *impaired glucose tolerance* (when a person has a two-hour glucose tolerance test result greater than 140 but less than 200 mg/dl). *Impaired glucose tolerance* means that blood sugar levels are worryingly high but not quite high enough to be classified as diabetes.

Diabetes is diagnosed when you've got a fasting blood sugar level equal to or greater than 126 mg/dl, or a two-hour glucose tolerance test level greater than or equal to 200 mg/dl – though some doctors have suggested lowering this upper limit to 180. Diabetes would be confirmed by a second test.

You can't cure diabetes, but you can reverse insulin resistance and reduce your risk of developing diabetes in the first place. Diabetes-prevention programmes have shown how effective diet and exercise can be in reversing insulin resistance and delaying and preventing the onset of diabetes.[7]

Some 40 to 50 per cent of women with PCOS experience weight problems, and research suggests that if you've got PCOS and are overweight you have a significantly increased risk of diabetes.[8] Although not everyone who becomes overweight will develop diabetes, insulin resistance tends to get worse when you gain weight.

So if you have PCOS and you're not overweight or insulin resistant, you don't have to read any more about diabetes, right? Wrong. It's important to point out here that, while overweight and insulin resistance do increase your diabetes risk significantly, studies show that the risk of diabetes is also increased in women with PCOS who are *not* overweight or insulin resistant.[9] This confirms the fact that PCOS is an independent risk factor for diabetes, and that all women with PCOS can benefit from taking action now to cut their risk of diabetes later.

Unfortunately, there are often few or no symptoms at all to alert you to the danger of diabetes – it doesn't happen overnight or over a few days; it develops slowly over time. This has helped to earn it the menacing nickname, 'the silent killer'. If you've got PCOS you should be tested regularly for diabetes and should also bear in mind that your risk increases significantly if, in addition to PCOS, you:

- are overweight
- have insulin resistance
- have high blood pressure
- have close relatives with diabetes

- have a diagnosis of hypertension
- are over 40
- have a history of gestational diabetes (diabetes that accompanies pregnancy)
- have a sedentary lifestyle.

WHAT SHOULD I WATCH OUT FOR?

With diabetes, the most recognizable symptom is fluid loss. Your body has to do something with all that extra glucose floating in your bloodstream, unable to get into the cells, and its solution is to eliminate the glucose in urine, which means tapping into your body's water supply. This sets the stage for the following symptoms:

- frequent need to use the restroom
- unusual thirst
- persistent fatigue for no apparent reason.

You may also notice that cuts and bruises are slow to heal, your vision is blurry, there is numbness or tingling in the hands and feet, reoccurring skin, gum or bladder infections and unexplained weight loss.

Unfortunately, many women with PCOS overlook their symptoms until it's too late and that's why, with our increased risk factor, it makes sense to be tested for diabetes every year, whether or not we notice any symptoms.

THE GOOD NEWS

The good news is that there's a lot you can do to reduce your risk of developing diabetes. Research shows that simple changes to your diet and lifestyle can prevent diabetes.[10] For example, a Finnish study showed that many people can significantly lower their diabetes risk

---

Will I get diabetes?

If you have PCOS, your risk of diabetes increases if:

- You have a parent, brother or sister with diabetes
- You have insulin resistance
- You have high blood pressure
- You have low levels of good cholesterol (high-density lipoproteins) or high levels of triglycerides (blood fats)
- You are 20 per cent or more above the recommended weight for your height
- You rarely, if ever, exercise
- You eat a lot of sugary, fatty, processed foods

The more of these that apply to you, the greater your chances of developing diabetes.

---

simply by making appropriate lifestyle changes, such as eating a low-fat, high-fibre diet and getting regular exercise.[11] Other studies[12] show that diet and lifestyle changes such as regular exercise, weight management,[13] a diet high in essential fatty acids[14] and low GI (glycaemic index) foods[15] can all reduce your risk.

Even better news

66 *When I was diagnosed with PCOS and diabetes it was like a double punch in the stomach — I was devastated. But now I've found a way of eating and living that can manage both conditions and I feel a lot more positive and in control. I'm living proof that with the right kind of diet, exercise and medication you don't have to endure poor health. Of course there are days when I wish I didn't have to be so careful with the food I eat, but then I think about how much better I feel when I eat healthily and get lots of exercise and I stop feeling sorry for myself.* 99

Jenna, 29

❝_I was diagnosed with diabetes at the same time that I was diagnosed with PCOS. I started medication and diet and lifestyle change right away and mercifully my PCOS symptoms are under control. It can seem really huge when life deals you the PCOS and diabetes card but life does go on and life can be good despite it all._ **❞**

Mary, 42

Research on PCOS shows clearly that the same diet and lifestyle changes that can prevent diabetes can also help ease common PCOS symptoms, such as irregular periods, acne, unwanted hair growth, weight gain and thinning hair.[16] If you can maintain appropriate blood sugar and insulin levels, you can significantly reduce your risk of developing diabetes while also minimizing the other effects of PCOS.

So seize this opportunity to take charge of your health, both now and in the future. Although having PCOS significantly increases your risk of developing diabetes, the diet and lifestyle changes recommended in our Protection Plan are designed to help you change the risk factors that are within your control, like diet, weight and exercise, and increase the likelihood that you'll live a healthier, happier life without ever getting this chronic disease.

REFERENCES

1. Fletcher, B. _et al._, 'Risk factors for type 2 diabetes mellitus', _J Cardiovasc Nurs_ 2002 Jan; 16 (2): 17–23; Pelusi, B. _et al._, 'Type 2 diabetes and the polycystic ovary syndrome', _Minerva Ginecol_ 2004 Feb; 56 (1): 41–51

2. Legro, R. _et al._, 'Prevalence and Predictors of Risk for Type 2 Diabetes Mellitus and Impaired Glucose Tolerance in Polycystic Ovary Syndrome: A Prospective, Controlled Study in 254 Affected Women', _J Clin Endocrinol Metab_ 1999; 84 (1): 165–9

3. De Leo, V. _et al._, 'Polycystic ovary syndrome and type 2 diabetes mellitus', _Minerva Ginecol_ 2004 Feb; 56 (1): 53–62

4. Solomon, C. _et al._, 'Long or irregular menstrual cycle as a marker for risk of type 2 diabetes mellitus', _J Am Med Assoc_ 2001 Nov; 286 (19): 2421–6

5. Ehrmann, D. A. *et al.*, 'Prevalence of impaired glucose intolerance and diabetes in women with polycystic ovary syndrome', *Diabetes Care* 1999; 22: 141–6
6. Goldstein, B. J. *et al.*, 'Insulin resistance: from benign to type 2 diabetes mellitus', *Rev Cardiovasc Med* 2003; 4 Suppl 6: S3–10
7. Molich, M. E. *et al.*, 'The diabetes prevention program and its global implications', *J Am Soc Nephrol* 2003 Jul; 14 (7 Suppl 2): S103–7
8. Ehrmann, D. A. *et al.*, 'Prevalence of impaired glucose intolerance and diabetes in women with polycystic ovary syndrome', *Diabetes Care* 1999: 22; 141–6
9. Dunaif, A. *et al.*, 'Beta cell dysfunction independent of obesity and glucose intolerance in the polycystic ovary syndrome', *J Clin Endocrinol Metab* 1996; 81: 942–7
10. Harris, S. B. *et al.*, 'Lifestyle interventions for type 2 diabetes. Relevance for clinical practice', *Can Fam Physician* 2003 Dec; 49: 1618–25: 'It is evident that supporting patients to make changes in their physical activity and dietary habits can prevent onset of type 2 diabetes.'
11. Eriksson, J. *et al.*, 'Prevention of Type II diabetes in subjects with impaired glucose tolerance: the Diabetes Prevention Study (DPS) in Finland. Study design and 1-year interim report on the feasibility of the lifestyle intervention programme', *Diabetologia* 1999 Jul; 42 (7): 793–801
12. Fujimoto, W. Y. *et al.*, 'Preventing diabetes – applying pathophysiological and epidemiological evidence', *Br J Nutr* 2000 Dec; 84 Suppl 2: S173–6
13. Steyn, N. P. *et al.*, 'Diet, nutrition and the prevention of type 2 diabetes', *Public Health Nutr* 2004 Feb; 7 (1A): 147–65
14. Das, U. N. *et al.*, 'Essential fatty acids in health and disease', *J Assoc Physicians India* 1999 Sep; 47 (9): 906–11
15. Rand, S. J. *et al.*, 'Diet in the prevention of diabetes and obesity in companion animals', *Asia Pac J Clin Nutr* 2003; 12 Suppl: S6
16. Norman, R. J. *et al.*, 'Polycystic ovary syndrome', *Med J Aust* 2004 Feb 2; 180 (3): 132–7; Norman, R. J. *et al.*, 'The role of lifestyle modification in polycystic ovary syndrome', *Trends Endocrinol Metab* 2002 Aug; 13 (6): 251–7

2 Obesity

If you're reading this because you have PCOS, chances are you've struggled with your weight, or are struggling still.

> 66 *I can't remember a time in my life when I wasn't on a diet. I've got PCOS and I'm overweight. My doctor has told me time and time again that it would help if I lost some weight, but whatever I do nothing shifts.* 99
>
> Pat, 34

> 66 *I've suffered with PCOS — acne, irregular periods, facial hair — for many years and wasn't surprised when my daughter was also diagnosed when she was 16 and the doctor put her on the Pill immediately. Apart from the pre-Pill menstrual irregularity she didn't seem to have any other symptoms. After college she went for a year to France to work as an English teacher. In her letters home she told me she had put on weight, but I didn't think much of it — who wouldn't put on weight in France? Nothing prepared me for the shock when I met her at the airport. I hardly recognized her. Her face was covered in acne and she'd put on nearly four stone.* 99
>
> Jane, 50

Being overweight is a common symptom of PCOS, and increasingly common full stop in Western society. Even being moderately overweight puts an undue stress on your back, legs and internal organs. But when overweight becomes obesity, you're setting yourself up for a whole load of other health problems, including diabetes, as we've seen in the previous chapter.

Obesity is quite simply an excess of body fat. Usually anyone who is 20 per cent over the normal weight for her age, sex, height and build is considered obese. Obesity increases your risk of diabetes because it increases your body's resistance to insulin – and insulin resistance also has a knock-on effect of increasing your ovaries' testosterone output, so makes PCOS symptoms worse, too.

Being obese also makes you more susceptible to infections (you might find you're always getting colds) and puts your heart and cardio-vascular system under strain, increasing your risk of heart disease and high blood pressure. It also puts your kidneys at risk of disease, as well as making it more likely you'll get arthritis from all the extra strain on your joints. And finally, being overweight or obese can cause psycho-logical suffering too, because our society tends to equate beauty, intel-ligence and even success with thinness.

WHAT CAUSES IT?

The most common causes of obesity are a poor diet and/or eating habits and a lack of exercise. If you don't get enough essential nutri-ents in your diet, your body can't burn fat easily and it can accumu-late in your body. Other problems that can contribute to obesity include diabetes, stress, eating disorders, an underactive thyroid, and hormonal problems like PCOS. Yes! Weight gain really is a symptom of PCOS, and you're not going mad if you've been trying to lose weight and finding it hard to shift. Perhaps you've been told by your doctor that you need to lose weight, and have felt very frustrated because you know you need to lose weight but, however hard you try, you can't. You hardly seem to eat anything but it makes no difference – the weight won't drop off.

Well, research shows that obesity is four times more likely in women who have PCOS and irregular periods than those without,[1] simply because our metabolism is wired differently.

The PCOS metabolism

Whether you've got PCOS or not, whenever you go on a diet and restrict calories your body eventually goes into starvation mode, conserving more energy and efficiently storing away the calories it does get, as fat reserves. The result is that, even though you're eating less, you're not losing weight.

If you've got PCOS, in addition to your body's typical reaction to restricted food intake, you've another hurdle to face: research suggests that women with PCOS store fat more efficiently and burn up calories more slowly than women who don't have PCOS.[2] 'Research has shown that overweight women with PCOS tend to eat fewer calories than women without,' says PCOS expert Dr Helen Mason, 'but they still struggle to lose weight. Even women with PCOS who are normal weight consider maintaining a normal weight as difficult a problem as those women who were overweight, showing that the issue of weight is a constant struggle for everyone.'

So why is this? It's partly down to having a sluggish PCOS metabolism, so here is the lowdown.

Your metabolic rate is the rate at which your body burns calories. The faster your metabolic rate, the more you can eat without putting on weight. The slower your metabolic rate, the more you need to watch your food intake. Metabolic rate is increased by any activity, including eating, and your body needs to use up energy to digest the food once you've eaten it. This energy-use after a meal is called *postprandial thermogenesis*. For most people, postprandial thermogenesis accounts for a good percentage of their calorie burning (you can often see someone's speeded up metabolism as they burn energy to digest their food if they get a red face or raised temperature after a meal) but studies show that postprandial thermogenesis in women with PCOS is significantly reduced.[3] So, if you have PCOS, you don't burn up as many calories after you eat a meal as someone who doesn't have PCOS. And the result is that you store more of the calories from the food you eat, which pushes up the likelihood of you gaining more weight.

And if you've got insulin resistance as well as PCOS, you also have to deal with the consequence of insulin preventing you from burning calories off. Insulin resistance causes your body's hormones to react in the opposite way to what you really want if you've got PCOS – that is, to store energy as fat rather than burn it off. According to Dr Legro in the *American Journal of Obstetrics and Gynecology*, women with PCOS show as much as a 40 per cent lower response to the hormones that trigger the breakdown of fat than women who don't have PCOS, whether or not the women with PCOS are obese.

WHAT'S MY OBESITY RISK?

As we've seen, not only does being overweight make you more likely to develop an increasing number and severity of PCOS symptoms, if you've got polycystic ovaries you're more likely to put on weight. Obesity is thought to be more likely in women who have PCOS than those without, with the latest studies showing that at least 50 per cent of women with PCOS are overweight or obese.[4]

With the odds stacked against us, it's small wonder that many of us comfort-eat or develop eating disorders in a desperate attempt to lose weight, but of course this isn't a solution. The havoc eating disorders can wreak on your health and well-being will eventually make your symptoms worse.

THE GOOD NEWS

What this book, and the majority of PCOS experts believe, is that diet and lifestyle changes are essential when it comes to managing the symptoms of PCOS and helping you lose or maintain weight.[5] And the same diet and lifestyle changes that can help you beat PCOS can also help you lose weight and reduce the long-term risk of PCOS- and obesity-related health problems at the same time.

Losing weight can be frustrating and stressful if you've got PCOS, but it's by no means impossible. The key is controlling your blood sugar and insulin levels – something people with diabetes have been doing for years. Our Protection Plan will show you that making specific changes in your diet and the way you eat will help you gain control of the situation, manage your weight, beat your symptoms, reduce the risk of diabetes, cardiovascular disease, high blood pressure and other PCOS-related complications and, last but by no means least, feel slimmer, fitter and better about yourself.

REFERENCES

1. Gambineri, A. *et al.*, 'Obesity and the polycystic ovary syndrome', *Int J Obes Relat Metab Disord* 2002 Jul; 26 (7): 883–96; Hartz, A. *et al.*, 'The association of obesity with infertility and related menstrual abnormalities in women', *Int J Obesity* 1979; 3: 57–73; Saheli, I. *et al.*, 'Pathogenesis of polycystic ovary syndrome: what's the role of obesity?', *Metabolism* 2004 Mar; 53 (3): 358–76; Draveka, I. *et al.*, 'Obesity is the major factor determining an insulin sensitivity and androgen production in women with anovulary cycles', *Bratisl Lek Listy* 2003; 104 (12): 393–9

2. Robinson, S. *et al.*, 'Postprandial thermogenesis is reduced in polycystic ovary syndrome and is associated with increased insulin resistance', *Clin Endocrinol (Oxf)* 1992 Jun; 36 (6): 537–43

3. Ibid.

4. Faloia, E. *et al.*, 'Body composition, fat distribution and metabolic characteristics in lean and obese women with polycystic ovary syndrome', *J Endocrinol Invest* 2004 May; 27 (5): 424–9

5. Richardson, M. R. *et al.*, 'Current perspectives in polycystic ovary syndrome', *Am Fam Physician* 2003 Aug 15; 68 (4): 697–704; Norman, R. J. *et al.*, 'The role of lifestyle modification in polycystic ovary syndrome', *Trends Endocrinol Metab* 2002 Aug; 13 (6): 251–7

3 Cardiovascular Disease

Researchers are now beginning to understand the close links between PCOS, cardiovascular disease and stroke.[1] In the past five years, several studies have suggested that women with PCOS have a significantly higher risk of developing cardiovascular disease than women without.[2]

WHAT IS IT?

Your cardiovascular system is made up of your heart and blood vessels. Blood is pumped by your heart and circulated throughout your body through your blood vessels to deliver oxygen, glucose and vital nutrients to your body's cells. The arteries that supply blood, nutrients and oxygen to your heart to keep it working properly are called coronary arteries. Changes in the health of your coronary arteries build up over many years, and can lead to a variety of heart conditions because the heart muscle has been starved of oxygen.

Common heart conditions

Irregularities of heart rhythm (arrhythmias)
Irregular beats can cause palpitations and breathlessness.

Heart failure
In this, the heart cannot pump enough blood well enough to keep up with the body's demands, leading to symptoms like breathlessness,

swollen ankles, coughing, fatigue and trouble breathing when lying down.

Arteriosclerosis

This is a clot in the blood vessel, the most common cause of obstruction. Arteriosclerosis is responsible for most deaths resulting from a heart attack or stroke.

Heart attack

If the coronary arteries that carry oxygen and nutrients to the heart muscle harden or narrow, the flow of oxygen-rich blood to the heart slows, causing chest pain (also called *angina*). The total blockage of an artery can result in a heart attack.

A heart attack may feel as if someone is applying intense pressure to your chest. The pain can last for several minutes, often extending to your shoulder, arm, neck or jaw. Other signs of a heart attack include sweating, nausea, vomiting, shortness of breath, dizziness, fainting, anxiety, difficulty swallowing, sudden ringing in the ears and loss of speech. The amount and type of chest pain differs from one person to another, and indeed from men to women. Some have an intense pain while others feel only a mild discomfort. Many mistake the signs of a heart attack for indigestion. Some have no symptoms at all, a situation referred to as a 'silent' heart attack.

Unfortunately, despite remarkable new technology for both diagnosis and treatment of heart disease, the first sign of it may be a life-threatening calamity. Disorders of the cardiovascular system are often far advanced when they make themselves known. An estimated 25 per cent of people who have heart attacks have had no previous symptoms of heart trouble.

So what does all this have to do with PCOS? Unfortunately, if you've got PCOS, your risk of heart disease is considerably higher than normal.[3] One major reason for this is that women with PCOS tend to have many of the risk factors already associated with heart disease. For example, women with PCOS have a greater tendency to be insulin resistant and overweight or obese – both major risk factors for heart disease. But there are other risks, too, according to research.[4] We've divided them into three categories:

1. those you can't change
2. those you can easily take steps to control
3. those which, though complicated by having PCOS, you can still take action to cut.

Factors you can't change

Heredity

If there's a family history of cardiovascular disease, the chances are the genes you've inherited from your parents could make you more liable to high cholesterol, obesity, high blood pressure or diabetes – all risk factors.

Age

Heart disease, like many other diseases, becomes more common the older we get. In the UK alone, over half of heart attacks occur in people over the age of 65.

The menopause

Although experts differ in their opinions, it's thought by many that a woman's risk of heart disease increases during and after the menopause, when levels of oestrogen fluctuate and decline. Oestrogen is supposed to have a protective effect on the heart.

While you can't change your age, family history or the fact that you'll go through the menopause, it can help to be informed so that you know you need to take extra care if any of these factors apply to you.

Factors you can control

Smoking

Cigarette smoking is strongly linked to the risk of cardiovascular disease. Chemicals in cigarette smoke are absorbed into your bloodstream from the lungs and circulate around the body, affecting every cell. These chemicals make the blood vessels narrow temporarily, and also cause blood cells to become stickier, increasing the risk of clots. Your risk may also increase if you live with someone who smokes, or spend time with smokers at work or in restaurants and bars. A recent study has highlighted the dangers of passive smoking, suggesting that it can increase your risk of heart disease by up to 50 per cent.[5] Professor Peter Whincup of the Department of Community Health Sciences at St George's Hospital Medical School in London, believes the study highlights the case for avoiding passive smoking: 'This study adds to the weight of evidence that passive smoking is harmful and strengthens the case for limiting exposure to passive smoking as much as we can.' Deborah Arnott, director of anti-smoking campaign group ASH, says: 'This important study provides yet more evidence of the serious health risks posed by second-hand smoke. It suggests that if you regularly breathe in other people's smoke at home or at work, your chances of getting heart disease may rise by more than a half.'

Stress

It's thought that stressful events, such as divorce or the death of a loved one, can flood your body with hormones such as adrenaline and cortisol which can weaken your cardiovascular system. Numerous studies[6] also suggest a link between stress and heart disease, and although some heart experts feel there is not yet 100 per cent conclusive proof that stress is linked to heart disease, many experts, such as Dr Dean Ornish, Clinical Professor of Medicine at the University of California, San Francisco, believe that the so-called type A personality – restless, highly driven workaholic type who can't relax and is prone to burn out – may have double the risk of high blood pressure and cardiovascular disease compared with the laid-back 'type B' personality.

Interestingly, a recent study on women with PCOS found that many couldn't process cortisol effectively, leading to increased circulation of this hormone in their bloodstream[7] – perhaps another reason why women with PCOS are at a higher risk of cardiovascular problems.

Physical inactivity

The evil twin of obesity is a sedentary lifestyle. About one-quarter of American women are considered 'couch potatoes', and in recent years scores of research studies have validated the positive effects of exercise on health. Exercise lowers the risk of chronic conditions ranging from heart disease to breast cancer and osteoporosis. The reason is simple: the more weight you carry, the harder your heart has to work. When you're overweight your heart actually has to push your blood through fat that lines and narrows your blood vessels, increasing the strain and wearing out the heart muscle much faster. Think of how your heart rate gets faster and faster as you struggle home with big bags of shopping – and then think about how any extra weight you're carrying has the same effect on a day-to-day basis. The closer to your normal Body Mass Index (BMI) range you are (see page 137), the better chance your heart has of being healthy.

High homocysteine levels

Over the last several years, many studies have confirmed that having high homocysteine levels increases your risk of artery disease[8] – in fact, some researchers now believe 30 per cent of cardiovascular disease is directly related to high levels of homocysteine. So what is it?

Homocysteine is an amino acid produced by your body when it's trying to process protein, but can't do it efficiently because you haven't enough essential nutrients to feed the biochemical processes needed, in particular vitamin B and folic acid. The typical Western diet of processed and fast foods, and high levels of stress lead to reduced levels of both B vitamins and folic acid.

Researchers have found, however, that you can significantly reduce your homocysteine levels by getting more folic acid, found in green leafy vegetables and wholegrains. Another bonus is that if you're planning a pregnancy, folic acid is essential to prevent neural tube defects such as spina bifida.

Factors complicated by PCOS

So we've looked at the heart disease risk factors that are beyond your control and within your control – but what about the other significant factors we know about, such as overweight and high cholesterol levels? These are more complex for you, simply because you have PCOS. Why? Because it seems that if you have PCOS your body is more likely to put on weight (as we have seen above), and researchers are also beginning to notice a connection between PCOS and hypertension and PCOS and high cholesterol levels.[9] And diabetes is also a risk factor for cardiovascular problems – and we've already seen the link to PCOS via insulin resistance.

Weight

An eight-year research study conducted by Jo Ann Manson, MD at Harvard Medical School found that up to 70 per cent of coronary artery disease in obese women was caused by their being overweight. The study also found that even for women who were only modestly overweight, the risk of developing coronary disease was up to 40 per cent higher than for women of normal weight. Excess weight is a risk factor because it raises the level of artery-clogging fat in the blood and increases the likelihood that a woman will develop high blood pressure or diabetes, in themselves factors in the increased risk of heart disease.

Diabetes

Good control of diabetes, with diet and lifestyle modification and medication if necessary, makes heart and circulation problems less common. Abnormal blood sugar levels can increase the risk of circulatory disorders, and poor control of diabetes can often result in very abnormal blood fats.

High blood cholesterol (over 200 mg/dl)

Cholesterol is not a hormone but a waxy, fat-like substance found in every cell. It's normally used by the body to form cell membranes and hormones. Cholesterol is carried throughout the body by lipoproteins. There are two types of lipoproteins: low-density lipoproteins (LDL) the so-called 'bad' cholesterol, and high-density lipoproteins (HDL), or 'good' cholesterol. LDL can mix with other substances to form plaque, which builds up in artery walls and causes dangerous blockages. HDL removes cholesterol from the blood and carries it to the liver to be metabolized. If your diet is too high in animal and dairy fats, the resulting plaque deposits will narrow the arteries, making it harder for blood to pump through. When plaque splits, a clot can form in the damaged area and blood supply can be cut off completely, causing severe chest pain and a heart attack. The higher your LDL cholesterol the higher your risk of cardiovascular disease, and women with PCOS tend to have higher-than-normal levels of LDL.[10] Cholesterol is measured in mg/dl – a measure of concentration using milligrams per decilitre in the blood.

High blood pressure (over 120/80)

The term 'blood pressure' actually refers to the pressure in the arteries that transport blood from your heart to the rest of your body. High blood pressure causes stress on the heart and circulation, and can lead to heart attacks and strokes. Research has shown that women with PCOS are four times more likely to get high blood pressure than women without,[11] partly due to the increased likelihood of women with PCOS to be overweight and/or having higher-than-normal cholesterol levels.

WHAT'S MY RISK?

'Women with PCOS may represent the largest female group at high risk for the development of early onset coronary artery disease,' says Evelyn Talbott, an associate professor of epidemiology at the University of Pittsburgh in Pennsylvania, whose study on the link between PCOS and heart disease was published in the November 2003 issue of *Arteriosclerosis, Thrombosis and Vascular Biology*. 'It's important for physicians

Will I get heart disease?

In addition to having PCOS:

- Do you smoke?
- Do you eat lots of meat and dairy products?
- Are you overweight?
- Do you rarely, if ever, exercise?
- Do you have insulin resistance or diabetes?
- Do you have high blood pressure?
- Do you have high cholesterol levels?
- Does heart disease run in your family?
- Is your life stressful?
- Do you have absent or irregular periods?
- Are you going through the menopause or have you been through it?

The more questions you've answered 'yes', the greater your chance of developing heart disease in your lifetime.

to recognize these symptoms as signs of a broader, chronic disorder and treat it accordingly, with early lifestyle interventions and/or medications that will reduce cardiovascular disease risks.'

66 *There's a history of heart disease in my family and my sister has dangerously high cholesterol and hypertension. So far I'm in the clear, but I've got PCOS and need to be extra vigilant. It's scary not so much for myself but because I've got three young kids and I want to be around to take care of them.* 99

Sonia, 40

66 *Acne, no periods and an expanding waistline – not something you'd automatically link with an increased risk for heart disease. When I was diagnosed with PCOS my doctor just put me on the Pill and never mentioned any thing else. If I hadn't done my research I'd still be none the wiser.* 99

Lucy, 33

❝I *was seven years old when my dad collapsed while playing football with my brother. He lived for two more years after that, but he never played football again. Watching someone you love die from heart disease is unbearably painful and something you never get over. I've got PCOS and abnormal cholesterol. I'm going to do all I can to make sure my partner and my loved ones never have to watch me suffer like that.* **❞**

Ann, 35

The harsh truth is that a PCOS diagnosis means that you already have a high number of risk factors for cardiovascular disease, which could result in heart attack or stroke.[12]

WHAT SHOULD I LOOK OUT FOR?

As we said earlier, heart or cardiovascular disease usually doesn't give you a warning before the symptoms strike – that's why it's good to know that you're at a higher risk with PCOS because it means you can work with your doctor to get regular tests for risk factors such as high cholesterol, and you can take charge of your lifestyle by stopping smoking, eating well and dealing with any overweight issues you have.

But even if your heart problems give you warning signs like angina, it's worth knowing that women's symptoms of heart disease are often different to men's[13] – because most studies looking at heart disease have excluded women, not only do we tend to think of heart disease as a male problem (even though it's currently the number-one cause of death in women over 50), we also tend to assume that the symptoms outlined in the studies are the ones we should be looking out for.

In actual fact, the typical warning signs mentioned above – angina or chest pains – often don't affect women. All too often the symptoms women do get are misdiagnosed as stress. This is because women's symptoms often seem unrelated to heart problems – fatigue, shortness of breath, jaw pain, neck pain, pain in the arms, back pain, sweating, fainting, palpitations, bloating, heartburn, vomiting, confusion and a feeling of heaviness between the breasts (this is how women experience chest pain; some describe it as a sinking feeling or a burning sensation, also described as an aching, throbbing or a squeezing sensation or a feeling that your heart is 'jumping' into your throat).

THE GOOD NEWS

All of this may sound scary, but heart disease is not an inevitable result of PCOS. Just as a tall person is more likely to bump her head on a door frame than a small one, so people with one or more risk factors are more likely to have a heart attack than those without any. Not every tall person hits her head on the door frame, and not everyone with risk factors gets heart disease.

Knowing the risks means you can take action now to protect yourself. Research clearly shows that preventive measures are really effective in cutting your risk of heart and cardiovascular disease.[14] You can stop smoking, you can reduce levels of bad cholesterol, you can avoid a couch potato lifestyle, you can combat hypertension by eating less salt and you can tackle obesity, even if you have to adjust the measures you take to ensure they're effective for you when you have PCOS. (For example, losing weight is possible when you have PCOS but you won't be able to follow what most people would think of as a 'diet' and expect to lose weight and keep it off; you need to eat right for PCOS to see results.)

Better still, by directly treating PCOS with diet and lifestyle changes, and medication if needed, you can bring your hormone levels into a normal range – not only minimizing or eliminating the symptoms and effects of PCOS, but also cutting the heart disease risk factors of obesity, high cholesterol and insulin levels.[15] Put simply, altering your diet and lifestyle can help you beat the symptoms of PCOS and cut your risk of heart disease at the same time.

REFERENCES

1. Christian, R. C. *et al.*, 'Prevalence and predictors of coronary artery calcification in women with polycystic ovary syndrome', *J Clin Endocrinol Metab* 2003 Jun; 88 (6): 2562–68

2. Wild, S. *et al.*, 'Cardiovascular disease in women with PCOS: A long-term follow up: A retrospective cohort study', *Clin Endocrinol (Oxf)* 52 (5) 2000: 595–600

3. Talbot, E. O. *et al.*, 'Cardiovascular risk in women with polycystic ovary syndrome', *Obstet Gynecol Clin North Am* 2001 Mar; 28 (1): 111–33

4. Read, A. *et al.*, 'A primary care intervention programme for obesity and coronary heart disease risk factor reduction', *Br J Gen Pract* 2004 Apr; 54 (501): 272–8; Giampaoeli, S. *et al.*, 'The global cardiovascular risk chart', *Ital Heart J* 2004 Mar; 5 (3 Suppl): 177–85; Hu, F. B. *et al.*, 'Overweight and obesity in women: health risks and consequences', *J Women's Health (Larchmt)* 2003 Mar; 12 (2): 163–72

5. Whincup, P. H. *et al.*, 'Passive smoking and risk of coronary heart disease and stroke: prospective study with cotinine measurement', *BMJ* Jun 2004; 10.1136/bmj.38146.427188.55.

6. Wolf, S. *et al.*, 'Predictors of myocardial infarction over a span of 30 years in Roseto, Pennsylvania', *Integr Physiol Behav Sci* 1992; 27 (3) 246–57

7. Tsilchorozidou, T. *et al.*, 'Altered cortisol metabolism in polycystic ovary syndrome: insulin enhances 5alpha-reduction but not the elevated adrenal steroid production rates', *J Clin Endocrinol Metab* 2003 Dec; 88 (12): 5907–13

8. Loverro, G. *et al.*, 'The plasma homocysteine levels are increased in polycystic ovary syndrome', *Gynecol Obstet Invest* 2002; 53 (3): 157–62

9. Cenk Sayin, N. *et al.*, 'Insulin resistance and lipid profile in women with polycystic appearing ovaries: implications with regard to polycystic ovary syndrome', *Gynecol Endocrinol* 2003 Oct; 17 (5): 387–96

10. Orio, F. Jr *et al.*, 'The cardiovascular risk of young women with polycystic ovary syndrome: an observational, analytical, prospective case-control study', *J Clin Endocrinol Metab* 2004 Aug; 89 (8): 3696–701. *Erratum* in: *J Clin Endocrinol Metab* 2004 Nov; 89 (11): 5621

11. Lefebvre, P. *et al.*, 'Long-term risks of polycystic ovaries syndrome', *Gynecol Obstet Fertil* 2004 Mar; 32 (3): 193–8

12. Macut, D. *et al.*, 'Cardiovascular risk in adolescent and young adult obese females with polycystic ovary syndrome (PCOS)', *J Pediatr Endocrinol Metab* 2001; 14 Suppl 5: 1353–59 (discussion page 1365); Christian, R. C. *et al.*, 'Prevalence and predictors of coronary artery calcification in women with polycystic ovary syndrome', *J Clin Endocrinol Metab* 2003 Jun; 88 (6): 2562–8;

Boulman, N. *et al.*, 'Increased C-reactive protein levels in the polycystic ovary syndrome: a marker of cardiovascular disease', *J Clin Endocrinol Metab* 2004 May 1; 89 (5): 2160–5; Taponen, S. *et al.*, 'Metabolic cardiovascular disease risk factors in women with self-reported symptoms of oligomenorrhea and/or hirsutism: Northern Finland Birth Cohort 1966 Study', *J Clin Endocrinol Metab* 2004 May; 89 (5): 2114–18; Talbot, E. O. *et al.*, 'Do women with polycystic ovary syndrome have an increased risk of cardiovascular disease? Review of the evidence', *Minerva Ginecol* 2004 Feb; 56 (1): 27–39

13. 'Diagnose this: the puzzle of pain. Which symptoms suggest a heart attack – and which don't?' *Heart Advis* 2003 Dec; 6 (12): 7

14. Whitlock, E. P. *et al.*, 'The primary prevention of heart disease in women through health behaviour change promotion in primary care', *Womens Health Issues* 2003 Jul-Aug; 13 (4): 122–41; Abraham, M. B. *et al.*, 'Preventing cardio-vascular events in patients with diabetes mellitus', *Am J Med* 2004 Mar 8; 116 Suppl 5A: 39S–46S

15. Ajossa, S. *et al.*, 'The treatment of polycystic ovary syndrome', *Minerva Ginecol* 2004 Feb; 56 (1): 15–26; Sukalich, S. *et al.*, 'Cardiovascular health in women with polycystic ovary syndrome', *Semin Reprod Med* 2003 Aug; 21 (3): 309–15

4 High Blood Pressure (Hypertension)

High blood pressure, or hypertension, is an extremely common form of cardiovascular disease – but also has lots of effects on its own, which is why we've given it its own chapter.

WHAT IS IT?

Everyone has blood pressure; it's essential to human life. It's the force exerted by your blood against the walls of your arteries as it's pumped by your heart through your body, delivering oxygen and nutrients to vital organs so they can keep functioning.

Blood pressure is measured using two numbers, read as a fraction. The top number represents the *systolic* pressure, or the force of blood as your heart beats; the bottom number, or *diastolic* pressure, reflects the force of blood as your heart relaxes between beats. Doctors measure blood pressure in millimetres of mercury (mm Hg).

The National Heart, Lung and Blood Institute defines ideal blood pressure as less than 120/80 mm Hg. High blood pressure begins at 140/90. If your reading falls anywhere between these two bench marks, or the top number is higher than it should be even though the bottom one is fine, you should pay close attention to it. The higher it climbs, the greater the health risks because your heart is working harder than it should to pump blood through narrowed or clogged arteries. This extra workload can cause your heart to enlarge and to struggle with getting blood around your body.

High blood pressure also causes stress on the heart and circulation, and, as most people are aware, causes strokes. Most strokes occur when a blood clot forms somewhere in the body and finds its way into an artery that feeds the brain, shutting off the flow of blood. But in the UK and US, high blood pressure is responsible for more heart attacks than strokes.

In addition to heart attacks and strokes, high blood pressure can also cause damage to your kidneys and your eyesight.

WHAT CAUSES IT?

Research shows that high blood pressure is associated with a number of risk factors, including age and heredity, and in general terms from a combination of stress, inadequate exercise and nutritional imbalance.[1]

Stress

Stress is one of the leading causes. When you're under stress, the hormone adrenaline is released and blood vessels narrow to allow a rapid transmission of oxygen and blood to the muscles and brain. Heart rate increases. All this is a natural response to an immediate or acute threat, but if the stress becomes repetitive or constant, the rise in blood pressure can end up being constant, increasing your risk of hypertension and a whole host of stress-related symptoms including headaches, exhaustion, mood swings and poor general health.

Diet

In areas of the world where salt intake is high there's also a tendency for high blood pressure to be prevalent. Salt has been shown to upset the delicate biochemical balance that exists in the body between sodium and potassium. These two minerals interact in a close manner in transporting nutrients to the cells and discharging waste from the cells, and anything that upsets their relationship alters the dynamics of cellular physiology. High intakes of sodium seem to have a depressing effect upon potassium levels, creating a tendency for extra cellular fluid to build up. This manifests in the body generally as swollen areas. If your tissues are swollen due to fluid build-up, this increases pressure on the tiny blood vessels throughout the tissues and can have a knock-on effect of raising blood pressure as a whole.

A lifetime of eating high-fat foods can also cause trouble, raising blood cholesterol which in turn leads to plaque build-up and narrowed arterial openings. And a diet high in sugar can also increase blood pressure, because excess sugar triggers the release of insulin – stimulating cholesterol production and increasing the likelihood of insulin resistance. (As many as 50 per cent of hypertensive people are also insulin resistant. Hypertension is also associated with most cases of diabetes.)

Overweight

Being overweight causes high blood pressure because the more weight you're carrying, the harder your heart has to work to pump the blood

---

Will I get high blood pressure?

In addition to PCOS:

- Do you eat a lot of salty foods?
- Do you eat a lot of sugary foods?
- Is your life stressful?
- Is there a family history of high blood pressure?
- Are you overweight?
- Do you smoke?
- Do you have insulin resistance/diabetes?
- Do you rarely, if ever, exercise?
- Do you have high cholesterol?

The more questions you've answered 'yes', the greater your chance of developing high blood pressure in your lifetime.

around your body and to supply all the extra tissues you're carrying with blood.

Smoking and alcohol

Smoking also has a direct and often dramatic effect upon blood pressure because the nicotine in cigarettes constricts your arteries.

Although a moderate intake of alcohol (1½ glasses of wine daily) can relax arteries, increase HDL and protect against hypertension and heart disease, excessive alcohol consumption can be harmful and cause long-term increases in blood pressure.

WHAT'S MY RISK?

"For months I put up with dizzy spells, insomnia, fatigue, headaches and a constant need to use the restroom, thinking it was all tied up with my PCOS. Was I shocked when my doctor diagnosed me with hypertension. I was only 22 and I didn't smoke, and although slightly overweight by no means obese. I had no idea.**"**

Jill, 27

"I've got PCOS and hypertension. Before giving me medication for hypertension my doctor gave me six months of diet and lifestyle change to see if that could reduce my blood pressure, but work was busy at the time and I didn't give it the attention it deserved. I'm now on medication for hypertension and my doctor says that it's probably lifelong. I've noticed that my sex drive seems to have dwindled since I've been on the medication and I need more sleep. My doctor says these are typical side-effects. I'd urge any woman with hypertension to do all she can to keep her blood pressure down with diet and lifestyle change. Medication may seem easiest in the short term, but in the long term it's not so hot.**"**

Barbara, 37

If you've got PCOS, your risk of high blood pressure is higher than that of a woman who hasn't got PCOS.[2] This is because many of the symptoms associated with PCOS, such as weight gain, high cholesterol and insulin resistance, are known to be risk factors for cardiovascular disease and its precursor, high blood pressure.

HOW DO I KNOW IF I HAVE IT?

Most women suffering from high blood pressure don't know it because the symptoms can often be chalked up to something else. It can sometimes produce symptoms such as ringing in the ears, frequent nosebleeds, headaches, dizziness, frequent urination, irritability, fatigue and aches and pains, but more often than not these are absent or so mild as to be taken as part of normal existence.

But if you've got PCOS you know there's a possibility of an increased risk and you have an early warning system that women without PCOS don't have. The longer the condition remains undiagnosed, the greater the chances of it causing damage – so it's important to make sure your blood pressure is monitored at regular intervals. This can be done by regular trips to a health professional, every six months, or by the use of simple self-monitoring equipment now available at relatively low cost. In many UK pharmacies you can also be tested for free.

THE GOOD NEWS

If high blood pressure has a bright side, it's that many of the risk factors – like obesity, poor diet and smoking as well as an inactive lifestyle – are relatively easy to control by self-help methods, and these self-help methods are also great for easing symptoms of PCOS. By making simple changes to your diet and lifestyle, you can beat PCOS symptoms and outsmart high blood pressure at the same time.[3]

REFERENCES

1. 'Most coronary heart disease traceable to four risk factors', *Heart Advis* 2003 Oct; 6 (10): 2

2. Richardson, M. R. *et al.*, 'Current perspectives in polycystic ovary syndrome', *Am Fam Physician* 2003 Aug 15; 68 (4): 697–704; Valasquez, E. *et al.*, 'Chronic complications of polycystic ovary syndrome', *Invest Clin* 2002 Sep; 43 (3): 205–13; Etling, M. W. *et al.*, 'Obesity, rather than menstrual cycle pattern or follicle cohort size, determines hyperinsulinaemia, dyslipidaemia and hypertension in ageing women with polycystic ovary syndrome', *Clin Endocrinol (Oxf)* 2001 Dec; 55 (6): 767–76

3. Turbas, B. *et al.*, 'Metabolic syndrome', *Acta Diabetol* 2003 Dec; 40 Suppl 2: S401–4

5 Syndrome X

Syndrome X, also referred to as metabolic syndrome, glucose intolerance, insulin resistance or pre-diabetes, is a term used to describe a set of factors found to increase the risk of a heart attack by 4 to 20 times.[1] These factors include elevated insulin levels (insulin resistance), central obesity (around the middle of the body – the classic 'apple' shape), high levels of blood fats – LDL (bad) cholesterol and triglycerides – and high blood pressure (hypertension). We'll discuss these in more detail a little later on in this chapter.

Both insulin resistance and Syndrome X increase your risk of heart disease and diabetes, and practically every other age-related disorder – including obesity, eye disease, cancer and Alzheimer's disease – because they affect, directly or indirectly, virtually every other disease process. In addition to physical symptoms, if you've got Syndrome X you may feel exhausted, spacey, depressed, irritable, tired or angry, often for no reason.

WHAT CAUSES IT?

Syndrome X is a disorder caused by your body's inability to make the most of the food you eat. Two of the key players in Syndrome X are substances that are regarded as essential for our health: glucose (blood sugar) and insulin. The foods we as a population now eat have made our levels of glucose and insulin spiral out of control. In other words, the typical Western diet creates levels of glucose and insulin that are too high for our bodies to cope with. In the correct amounts, glucose and insulin help our bodies metabolize food and burn energy and fat, but in high doses they accelerate the ageing process, confuse the metabolism and encourage the development of Syndrome X.

Syndrome X is caused primarily by a diet high in sugary foods such as refined carbohydrates (sugary cereals, muffins, bread, biscuits, cakes, pastas, etc.). These refined carbohydrates not only raise glucose and insulin to unhealthy levels but also fail to supply the many nutrients the body needs to protect us from disease.

Will I get Syndrome X?

In addition to PCOS:

- Is your diet high in sugar and refined carbohydrates?
- Do you have insulin resistance/diabetes?
- Are you overweight – with most of that excess weight around your stomach?
- Do you have high cholesterol?
- Do you have high blood pressure?
- Do you have a family history of diabetes/heart disease?
- Do you have absent or irregular periods?

The more questions you've answered 'yes', the greater your chance of developing Syndrome X in your lifetime.

WHAT'S MY RISK?

66 *I was diagnosed with PCOS when I was 31; by the time I hit 40 my weight had crept up to 250 pounds [17½ stone] – and I'm only 5'4! – and my blood pressure was a dangerously high 145/95. With abnormal cholesterol readings on top of that, I was a prime candidate for a heart attack. To cap it all, my blood sugar levels were also high, so I was well on the way to developing diabetes.* **99**

Sue, 42

Many women with PCOS have features of Syndrome X, in particular insulin resistance and obesity.[2] As we've seen, it's estimated that at least half of the women with PCOS have detectable insulin resistance and weight-management problems – and often this excess weight tends to cluster around the waist. Studies show a tendency for women with PCOS to put weight on around the waist rather than the hips – making for an apple shape rather than a pear shape.[3] Experts believe that gaining weight around the middle is associated with a higher risk of Syndrome X.[4] There is no definitive evidence about why 'being an apple' carries with it more health risks than 'being a pear', but it's believed that it may be due to the way the body processes fat stored in different parts of the body. Fat around the tummy is constantly being broken down and circulated around the body (unlike fat around the hips), and higher levels of circulating fat increase the risk of heart disease, narrowing of the arteries, high blood pressure, diabetes and certain cancers.

Am I an apple or a pear?

This is simple: Measure your waist and the widest part of your hips. If your waist measurement is higher, you're an apple. If your hip measurement is higher, you're a pear.

Alongside this, however, there are also ratios to be aware of. Divide your waist measurement by your hip measurement. According to the US National Institute of Diabetes and Digestive and Kidney Diseases, women with a waist-to-hip ratio of greater than 0.8 are at greater risk of diabetes, high blood pressure and heart disease.

In addition to elevated insulin levels and central obesity, many women with PCOS also have the two other significant Syndrome X risk factors: high levels of blood fats (cholesterol and triglycerides) and high blood pressure.[5]

It would seem that a woman with PCOS has all the risk factors for Syndrome X, which begs the question: Is Syndrome X actually just a cardiologist's view of what a gynaecologist would call PCOS?

Current thinking suggests that the two are slightly different (see below), but as more research is done, they may turn out to be different views of the same condition after all – not least because a couple of studies[6] looking at male relatives of women with PCOS found they were more likely to have insulin resistance and abnormal blood fat profiles as well as premature baldness, showing that the metabolic aspects of PCOS can cross genders, while the gynaecological aspects restrict themselves to women simply because men can't develop them.

'There are strong similarities between the conditions,' says PCOS expert Dr Adam Balen, Professor of Reproductive Medicine and Surgery at Leeds General Infirmary, 'but they aren't the same – it's more complicated than that.' More research needs to be done, but for now the difference between PCOS and Syndrome X lies in the fact that in Syndrome X there's always insulin resistance, elevated insulin production and inefficient glucose metabolism (promoting increased blood fats, blood pressure and obesity). So if you've got insulin resistance, high blood fats, high blood pressure and are overweight, you definitely have Syndrome X. PCOS, on the other hand, isn't so easy to define. For now, research is primarily focused on whether PCOS is an early sign of or a risk factor for Syndrome X.[7]

THE GOOD NEWS

Studies show that the safest and most effective therapy to reduce the risk of Syndrome X is a healthy diet along with regular exercise and weight loss.[8] And the same healthy diet and lifestyle modifications can significantly improve the symptoms of PCOS.[9]

The message is clear: Just as you don't have to put up with the symptoms of PCOS destroying the quality of your life, you don't have to accept Syndrome X as an inevitable part of PCOS. There are things you can do to reverse the syndrome if you've got it – and things you can do to stop PCOS from developing into Syndrome X.

REFERENCES

1. Nelson, M. R. *et al.*, 'Managing "metabolic syndrome" and multiple risk factors', *Aust Fam Physician* 2004 Apr; 33 (4): 201–5
2. Ehrmann, D. A. *et al.*, 'Insulin resistance and polycystic ovary syndrome', *Curr Diab Rep* 2002 Feb; 2 (1): 71–6
3. Evans, D. J. *et al.*, 'Relationship of androgenic activity to body fat topography, fat cell morphology and metabolic aberrations in premenopausal women,' *J Clin Endocrinol Metab* 57 (1983) 304–10
4. Wong, S. *et al.*, 'Abdominal adipose tissue distribution and metabolic risk', *Sports Med* 2003; 33 (10): 709–26
5. Strowitski, L. *et al.*, 'Body fat distribution, insulin sensitivity, ovarian dysfunction and serum lipoproteins in patients with polycystic ovary syndrome', *Gynecol Endocrinol* 2002 Feb; 16 (1): 45–51; Richardson, M. R. *et al.*, 'Current perspectives in polycystic ovary syndrome', *Am Fam Physician* 2003 Aug 15; 68 (4): 697–704
6. Duskova, M. *et al.*, 'What may be the markers of the male equivalent of polycystic ovary syndrome?', *Physiol Res* 2004; 53 (3): 287–94
7. Legro, R. S. *et al.*, 'Polycystic ovary syndrome and cardiovascular disease: a premature association?', *Endocr Rev* 2003 Jun; 24 (3): 302–12; Svanina, A. *et al.*, 'Metabolic aspects of the polycystic ovary syndrome', *Vnitr Lek* 2002 Dec; 48 (12): 1142–6; Botella, L. J. *et al.*, 'Metabolic syndrome X in women', *An R Acad Nac Med (Madr)* 2000; 117 (2): 317–27; discussion 327–30
8. Erbas, T. *et al.*, 'Metabolic syndrome', *Acta Diabetol* 2003 Dec; 40 Suppl 2: S401–4
9. Glueck, C. J. *et al.*, 'Incidence and treatment of metabolic syndrome in newly referred women with confirmed polycystic ovarian syndrome', *Metabolism* 2003 Jul; 52 (7): 908–15

6 Cancer

We know this word often makes people panic, but we also get asked a lot about whether PCOS has links with hormonal cancers.

We're happy to report that more research than ever is now being done into many aspects of PCOS, that are helping to build up a clearer picture of its effects on hormonal-related cancers.

WHAT IS CANCER?

Cancer happens when cells escape the normal mechanisms that control their growth and replication, so that they speed up and multiply in an out-of-control way. When these cells start to invade surrounding tissues, they are called malignant because their accelerated growth creates a tumour which can cause damage to the body.

WHAT CAUSES IT?

This is the million-dollar question – and one which research scientists all over the world are working hard to answer. What we do know is that it's unlikely that there's a single cause – although researchers are still looking to find one.

It's most likely that cancer involves a number of factors beginning with a genetic predisposition which alters some cells or your body's response to the environment. There then seems to be a long-term chronic 'promoter' which triggers the cancer – for example, with lung cancer the promoter may be smoking, with breast cancer the promoter may be levels of oestrogens that are too high. But the reason why a cell becomes cancerous is still a mystery. As a spokesperson at Cancer Research UK has put it, 'Cancers develop because of a complicated interaction between our genes, our environment and chance.'

WHAT'S MY RISK?

'There are numerous case reports in the literature on the association of PCOS and the development of endometrial cancer in young women and women over 40,' says PCOS expert Professor Gabor Kovacs from Monash Medical School, Box Hill Hospital, Melbourne, Australia. Research does suggest that women with PCOS of all ages have an increased risk of endometrial cancer.[1] It's not hard to see why, as the risk factors for endometrial cancer include irregular periods, obesity and family history[2] – all familiar features of PCOS. It's also thought that women with PCOS may have an increased risk of ovarian and breast cancer.[3] Let's take a closer look at each of these cancers in turn.

ENDOMETRIAL HYPERPLASIA – A WARNING SIGN FOR ENDOMETRIAL CANCER

If you have PCOS and you don't have regular periods, your body isn't shedding and replacing your womb lining (endometrium) every month. Normally, under the influence of oestrogen the cells of the uterine lining multiply, usually in the first half of the menstrual cycle before ovulation. At ovulation, the hormone progesterone is released, eventually triggering the shedding of the womb lining (if there is no pregnancy) in readiness for another cycle. If you don't ovulate, and therefore don't release progesterone, the unopposed oestrogen carries on sustaining the growing womb lining and a build-up of the endometrium occurs. The more time that passes without a period, the more build-up occurs. Left unchecked, this may result in an overgrowth of the endometrium – this is called *hyperplasia*.

What should I look out for?

The earliest signs of endometrial development may be erratic and heavy bleeding. While certainly not cancer, hyperplasia is moving in that direction and should be considered a warning sign. There are two main types of hyperplasia:

1. simple hyperplasia, which carries a risk of developing endometrial cancer
2. hyperplasia with atypia (a medical term for the presence of abnormal, pre-cancerous cells) – this holds a much higher risk – 50 per cent or greater.

The main thing to take away from this is that if you're not having at least four periods a year, you should talk to your doctor about inducing them to reduce your risk.

66*I hate doctors, always have. Every time I got a letter suggesting I go for a smear test I would file it somewhere I knew I would never find it. When I went down with a terrible bout of flu which seemed to drag on for weeks I was forced to see the doctor and he asked me some questions about my health. He asked me when I'd had my last period and I told him I couldn't remember. He urged me to have a smear test and I reluctantly agreed. A few weeks later I was diagnosed with PCOS and also got an abnormal smear test result. It was treated and I'm in the clear, but it was a big lesson to me and I'm going to make sure I'm tested regularly from now on.* **99**

Victoria, 28

UTERINE AND ENDOMETRIAL CANCER

If left untreated, endometrial hyperplasia can develop into cancer of the uterus or endometrium. The US Centers for Disease Control, in their *Cancer and Steroid Hormone* study, reported that women who had a history of PCOS and irregular periods had a five-fold increase in endometrial cancer.[4]

The good news

The good news is that you can reduce your risk of endometrial hyperplasia, uterine or endometrial cancer, and beat symptoms of PCOS at the same time, with healthy diet and lifestyle changes designed to balance your hormones and regulate your menstrual cycle. If you get your hormones back in balance, you'll be more likely to have periods, and more able to lose or manage your weight.

It's also important that you see your doctor for a complete gynaecological exam each year, especially if your periods are irregular or nonexistent. Why? Almost all endometrial cancers are found early in their development, with proper check-ups, often because of their association with abnormal vaginal bleeding — and once it has been diagnosed the chances of recovery are good. Studies show that the cure rate is high regarding endometrial cancer in women with PCOS, though this cure often involves hysterectomy.[5] So any steps you can take to reduce the risk of developing it in the first place will be well worth while.

OVARIAN CANCER

Many women with PCOS worry about ovarian cancer when they see ultrasound scan results that show enlarged ovaries and 'cysts'. But what are the true risks?

In the US, ovarian cancer is the sixth most common cancer in women and the leading cause of death from what is known as 'gynaecological' cancer. In the UK it is the fourth most common cancer for women, with

---

PCOS and the birth control pill

The close link between PCOS and endometrial cancer underscores the need for preventive screening through regular gynaecological check-ups in women with PCOS. With this understanding it becomes apparent that treating irregular menstrual cycles is more than a matter of convenience. If you have PCOS, inducing regular, cyclic shedding of the uterine lining will actually lower your risk of developing endometrial cancer. That's why the most commonly used strategy to treat PCOS and induce regular menstrual cycles is the birth control Pill. This may be the choice you and your doctor feel is the right one for you.

But to make the most of the benefits the Pill can offer you, do bear in mind that there are health risks associated with being on it and being overweight, such as blood clots and high blood pressure, so you may need to work hard at getting to a healthy weight before your doctor will prescribe it, and you should make sure you maintain a healthy weight while you're taking it. The synthetic oestrogens in the Pill can also increase the drive towards weight gain and insulin resistance, both of which are associated with a worsening of PCOS symptoms over the long term.[6] Not to mention the fact that some studies suggest the Pill may leach valuable supplements and nutrients as well as alter your vitamin and mineral levels and increase levels of bad cholesterol.[7]

So, once again it's really important to use PCOS treatment responsibly with advice from your doctor, and to make healthy diet and lifestyle changes, with or without medication, to ensure you get the benefits with the least risk of any side-effects.

---

around 4,700 deaths a year. At birth a woman has a one in 70 chance of developing ovarian cancer later in life; most cancers occur in the post-menopausal years. A major problem comes from the silent progression of ovarian cancer and its vague, easily misdiagnosed symptoms such as abdominal fullness, alteration in bowel function and fatigue.

What causes it?

Ovarian cancer rates tend to go down for women who have given birth a number of times and/or who have been on the contraceptive Pill for many years, because both provide a protective 'time off' from ovulation. The theory of incessant ovulation and exposure to high levels of oestrogen prior to ovulation has been put forward to explain the development of ovarian cancer; if it's true that the number of ovulations predicts the risk of cancer, then an early puberty and late menopause would place a woman at increased risk.

There's not, however, universal agreement on the ovulation-and-oestrogen theory. It has been suggested that androgens may be the culprits, which isn't good news if you've got PCOS. Other theories include exposure to environmental toxins or long-term use of fertility drugs, but to date no theory has received confirmation or universal support.

What's my risk?

As we've seen, there's uncertainty about what actually causes ovarian cancer, although some studies do suggest a modestly increased risk if you've got PCOS.[8] At the same time, however, these studies point out the complexity of the PCOS association with other possible cancer risk factors such as obesity, insulin resistance and hormonal imbalance.

The good news

With no certain knowledge about the real connection between risk factors of PCOS and ovarian cancer, you can at least feel comforted that PCOS can act as an early warning system. The diagnosis of ovarian cancer is easily made by ultrasound scan, and as ultrasound screening is routinely used to diagnose and monitor PCOS, signs of ovarian cancer can be detected early enough to make a difference. And, although the relationship between a healthy diet and prevention of ovarian cancer has yet to be confirmed, the benefits of a healthful diet, exercise and weight management for cancer prevention in general is well known, so you can take control of your health in this way.

BREAST CANCER

We all know our breasts respond to hormonal surges and drops, as confirmed by the changes our breasts undergo (increased tenderness, swelling) during our menstrual cycle or as a result of our PCOS. Recent studies that have shown an increased risk of breast cancer in women taking HRT have also revealed that the breast tissues are directly affected by hormonal balance. This has led to many women with PCOS wondering if they're at an increased (or even decreased) risk of breast cancer if they're not ovulating.

What are the facts?

Your breasts depend on hormonal stimulation for their development and function, but while we know some of the other risk factors for breast cancer (see below), we don't know them all.

What risks do we know about?

A family history of breast cancer is associated with an increased risk, and obviously this is something you can't change. But there are other factors within your control. For instance, many researchers believe a high-fat diet increases the production of the kind of oestrogens that can trigger cancer.[9]

In the same way as there is 'good' and 'bad' cholesterol, some researchers now believe that the body's natural oestrogen, oestradiol, can be converted into two distinct products that are similar in structure but act quite differently. One product is thought to protect against breast cancer, while the other does not. This has led some researchers to believe that this 'bad' oestrogen is overproduced in women exposed to high levels of xenoestrogens – the synthetic or man-made oestrogens in the environment that come from plastics, pesticides, chemical fertilizers and even the parabens in cosmetics. The parabens link has been hotly disputed and gave rise to rumours about anti-perspirants containing aluminium causing breast cancer. While a recent study showed there is possibly a link between the two,[10] more research is being done.

Obesity is definitely a risk.[11] An inactive lifestyle is, too – because not only does lack of physical exercise encourage obesity, it also prevents the beneficial effects exercise has on decreasing the type of oestrogens in the body that are related to cancer.

It's also thought that a high intake of alcohol increases the risk, as alcohol alters the body's hormone balance by making the liver less able to detoxify some substances that contribute to breast cancer.[12] And some new studies suggest that smoking may raise breast cancer risk as well.[13]

So if you've got PCOS, how do these risks stack up? Several studies have suggested that women with PCOS may have an increased risk due to the obesity link and hormonal fluctuations that can lead to unopposed oestrogen in the body and irregular or absent periods when you don't ovulate.[14,15] More research needs to be done, but for now we need to assume that the risk of breast cancer could be increased for women with PCOS.

This means taking preventative measures – the obvious ones, as for all these PCOS risks, are stopping smoking if you're a smoker, drinking moderately, eating healthily and getting more active.

On top of these, you'll be pleased to hear that the lifestyle and diet changes that can ease PCOS symptoms exactly match those recommended for the prevention of breast cancer.[16] Once again, PCOS acts as an early warning system, giving us both a reason and the motivation to self-examine regularly, to consult our doctors about regular screening and to take the necessary preventative measures with positive diet and lifestyle changes.

REFERENCES

1. Gregorini, S. D. *et al.*, 'Endometrial carcinoma with polycystic ovaries: report to two cases in women younger than 40 years', *Medicina (B Aires)* 1997; 57 (2): 209–12; Dahlgren, E. *et al.*, 'Endometrial carcinoma; ovarian dysfunction – a

risk factor in young women', *Eur J Obstet Gynecol Reprod Biol* 1991; 41: 143–50

2. Gerber, J. *et al.*, 'The risk factors of endometrial cancer', *Ginekol Pol* 2001 Dec; 72 (12A): 1418–22

3. Balen, A. *et al.*, 'Polycystic ovary syndrome and cancer', *Hum Reprod Update* 2001 Nov-Dec; 7 (6): 522–5

4. Hardiman, P. *et al.*, 'Polycystic ovary syndrome and endometrial carcinoma', *Lancet* 2003 May 24; 361 (9371): 1810–12; Erratum in *Lancet* 2003 Sep 27; 362 (9389): 1082

5. Balen, A. *et al.*, 'Polycystic ovary syndrome and cancer', *Hum Reprod Update* 2001 Nov-Dec; 7 (6): 522–5

6. British Medical Association, *Official Guide to Medicine and Drugs* (Dorling Kindersley, 1998): 147

7. Sutterlin, M. W. *et al.*, 'Serum folate and vitamin B_{12} levels in women using modern oral contraceptives (OC) containing 20 microg ethinyl estradiol', *Eur J Obstet Gynecol Reprod Biol* 2003 Mar 26; 107 (1): 57–61; Tyrer, L. B., 'Nutrition and the pill', *J Reprod Med* 1984 July; 29 (7): Suppl 547–50; Theuer, R. *et al.*, 'Effect of oral contraceptive agents on vitamin and mineral needs; a review', *J Reprod Med* 1972 Jan; 8 (1)

8. Spremovi, R. S. *et al.*, 'The polycystic ovary syndrome associated with ovarian tumor', *Srp Arh Celok Lek* 1997 Nov-Dec; 125 (11–12): 375–7

9. Walker, M. R. *et al.*, 'Breast cancer – can risks really be lessened?', *Eur J Cancer Prev* 2000 Aug; 9 (4): 223–9

10. Harvey, P. W. *et al.*, 'Endocrine disrupters and human health: could oestrogenic chemicals in body care cosmetics adversely affect breast cancer incidence in women?', *J Appl Toxicol* 2004 May-Jun; 24 (3): 167–76

11. Su, F. H. *et al.*, 'Overweight and obesity in women: health risks and consequences', *J Women's Health (Larchmt)* 2003 Mar; 12 (2): 163–72

12. Benassi, B. *et al.*, 'Alcohol, genome instability and breast cancer', *Asia Pac J Clin Nutr* 2004; 13 (Suppl): S55

13. Manjer, J. *et al.*, 'Smoking is associated with postmenopausal breast cancer in women with high levels of estrogens', *Int J Cancer* 2004 Nov 1; 112 (2): 324–8

14. Wild, S. *et al.*, 'Long-term consequences of polycystic ovary syndrome: results of a 31-year follow-up study', *Hum Fertil (Camb)* 2000; 3 (2): 101–5

15. Hunter, M. D. *et al.*, 'Polycystic Ovary Syndrome: It's not just infertility', *American Family Physician*, American Academy of Family Physicians, Sep 1, 2000

16. Hu, F. B. *et al.*, 'Overweight and obesity in women: health risks and consequences', *J Women's Health* (Larchmt) 2003 Mar; 12 (2): 163–72

7 Bone Health

You may think that you only need to worry about osteoporosis when you're over 50, or that as long as you get enough calcium in your diet, bone health won't be an issue. But it's worth knowing that having PCOS can actually increase your risk, as yo-yo and crash dieting are often indicated in its development and many of us, struggling with our weight, have spent years giving ourselves poor nutrition.

WHAT IS OSTEOPOROSIS?

Osteoporosis is a disease of the skeleton in which the amounts of calcium present in the bones slowly decreases to the point that bones become brittle and prone to fracture. It currently affects 9 million Americans, while another 16 million are at high risk for fractures due to low body density. There are no warning signs for this crippling disease – often the first indication that there's a weakening of the bones is a fracture that occurs after a minor fall. Hip fractures and their complications result in the deaths of more women than deaths from cervical, ovarian and uterine cancer combined.

WHAT CAUSES IT?

Risk increases with age as bone begins to lose density after the mid-thirties. Women who are thin with a small-boned frame are at greater risk because they have less bone mass in the first place. Genetics plays its part here, as 80 per cent of bone density is genetically determined. Other factors that increase risk include a diet low in calcium, fruits and vegetables, unhealthy habits such as smoking, alcohol consumption and drinking too many fizzy drinks, and an inactive lifestyle – exercise strengthens not just muscle but bones, too. And because of the natural decline in oestrogen at the menopause (decreasing levels of oestrogen hasten bone loss), one-third of all women develop osteoporosis after the menopause.

Will I get osteoporosis?

In addition to PCOS:

- Are you constantly dieting?
- Are you small boned or thin?
- Do you smoke?
- Do you drink?
- Have you had an eating disorder?
- Do you rarely, if ever, exercise?
- Is there a family history of osteoporosis?
- Are you approaching or going through the menopause?

The more questions you've answered 'yes', the greater your chance of developing osteoporosis in your lifetime.

WHAT'S MY RISK?

66 *Since the age of about 12 I've been dieting. I cut out meat and dairy foods altogether and, looking back, don't quite know how I survived. I hardly ate a thing. I didn't have periods either and was diagnosed with PCOS and put on the Pill by my doctor. My starvation years continued until I went to college and suddenly discovered food, friendship and fun. I put on a lot of weight in the first two terms, but I hated the way I looked and dieted strictly again. The following year the weight crept back and I dieted it away again. This yo-yo dieting went on for years until my early thirties when I had a fall and broke my arm while playing netball.*

*It took ages and ages to heal, and concerned doctors gave me a scan. I
had the bone density of a 60 year old.* **99**

Debbie, 35

At first glance it might seem that women with PCOS don't have to worry
about an increased risk of osteoporosis. Some experts believe that PCOS
may even have a protective effect on bone health due to the increased
weight and higher-than-normal levels of bone-protecting oestrogen
associated with PCOS.[1] But this potentially protective effect can be offset
by constant attempts to lose weight using unhealthy diets. Studies have
shown how important a healthy, nutritious diet is for bone health and
how poor eating habits can increase the risk of osteoporosis.[2]

Research also suggests[3] that although PCOS doesn't cause eating
disorders, as many as 60 per cent of sufferers may have disordered
eating patterns such as bulimia.[4] And when eating patterns are
disturbed and diet is poor, the bones just aren't getting the nutrients
they need to stay healthy and strong.

THE GOOD NEWS

If you've got PCOS and you know that your diet has not been as healthy
as it could, or you've jumped from drastic diet to drastic diet with
bingeing and comfort eating in between, the good news is that osteoporosis is not an inevitable part of ageing. Weight-bearing exercise, a
healthy, calcium-rich diet, and once again cutting out smoking and too
much alcohol will all help to protect your bones. Supplementing with
extra calcium if you're in your forties or have been eating unhealthily
for many years is also wise.

REFERENCES

1. Lupoli, G. *et al.*, 'Gonadotropin-releasing hormone agonists administration in
    polycystic ovary syndrome. Effects on bone mass', *J Endocrinol Invest* 1997 Sep;
    20 (8): 493–6

2. Seidenfeld, S. E. *et al.*, 'Impact of anorexia, bulimia and obesity on the gynecologic health of adolescents', *Am Fam Physician* 2001 Aug 1; 64 (3): 445–50; Pentice, A. *et al.*, 'Diet, nutrition and the prevention of osteoporosis', *Public Health Nutr* 2004 Feb; 7 (1A): 227–43; Turner, L. W. *et al.*, 'Changes in behavior and behavioral intentions among middle-aged women: results from an osteoporosis prevention program', *Psychol Rep* 2003 Oct; 93 (2): 521–6; Zborowski, J. *et al.*, 'Polycystic ovary syndrome, androgen excess, and the impact on bone', *Obstet Gynecol Clin North Am* 2001 Mar; 28 (1): 135–51

3. Michaelmore, K. F. *et al.*, 'Polycystic ovaries and eating disorders: Are they related?', *Hum Reprod* 2001 Apr; 16 (4): 765–9

4. Jahanfar, S. *et al.*, 'Bulimia nervosa and polycystic ovary syndrome', *Gynecol Endocrinol* 1995 Jun; 9 (2): 113–17; McCluskey, S. *et al.*, 'Polycystic ovary syndrome and bulimia', *Fertil Steril* 1991 Feb; 55 (2): 287–91

5. Rotterdam ESHRE/ASRM-Sponsored PCOS Consensus Workshop Group, 'Revised 2003 consensus on diagnostic criteria and long-term health risks related to polycystic ovary syndrome', *Fertil Steril* 2004 Jan; 81 (1): 19–25; Hippelainen, M. *et al.*, 'Polycystic ovarian syndrome is a health risk', *Duodecim* 2002; 118 (10): 981–3; Kelly, C. J. *et al.*, 'The long-term health consequences of polycystic ovary syndrome', *BJOG* 2000 Nov; 107 (11): 1327–38

6. Ajossa, A. *et al.*, 'The treatment of polycystic ovary syndrome', *Minerva Ginecol* 2004 Feb; 56 (1): 15–26

8 Take Heart

Even though it's hard to think that it may happen to you, the harsh truth is that PCOS does carry with it serious long-term health risks you can't afford to ignore. The good news is that there's a lot you can do right now to prevent the long-term complications and avoid becoming a victim of the serious health risks associated with PCOS.

While it may be sobering news to learn that PCOS puts you at risk of these serious conditions, you'll also have seen that diet and lifestyle can have massively positive effects in preventing you from getting these conditions. And the best news of all is that your diet and lifestyle are within your control, which means your risk of developing some of the serious complications associated with PCOS are, too.

You may have noticed that many of the risk factors and diet and lifestyle recommendations for diabetes, heart disease and other PCOS complications were similar. Moreover, these lifestyle changes are also the ones recommended to keep PCOS symptoms in check. The facts show that exercise, weight-management and healthy eating not only ease day-to-day PCOS symptoms but also provide powerful protection against poor health in the future. And the wonderful thing about all this is that diet and lifestyle changes are within your control. In partnership with a good healthcare professional who can monitor your risks and give you regular check-ups, you have a great chance to fight back. You really can challenge PCOS and stack the odds in your favour by changing your lifestyle for the better and protecting your long-term health.

Don't let PCOS, and the health risks associated with it, make you feel helpless. Instead let PCOS remind you that you do have power over your health. Our Protection Plan in Part Two is designed to help you take that power and use it.

Part Two
Your Protection Plan

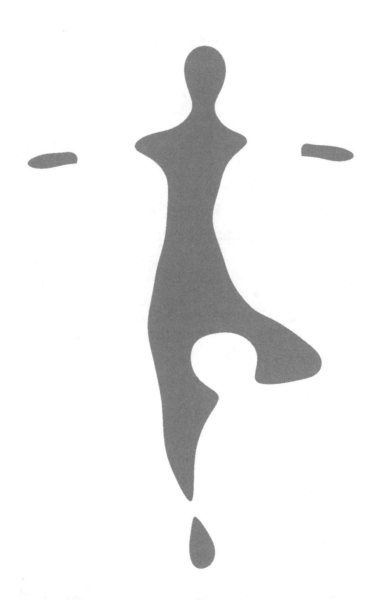

9 You Are What You Eat

You may already have noticed how the symptoms of PCOS and the long-term health risks associated with them are interrelated, with knock-on effects on each other. For example, obesity, a common symptom of PCOS, increases the likelihood of high blood pressure, insulin resistance, diabetes and heart disease. Insulin resistance, for its part, increases the likelihood of high blood pressure, obesity and diabetes, and so on.

While this might at first seem frustrating, it's actually a gift in some ways, too – because by taking measures that tackle one of these inter-related risks, you'll have a positive knock-on effect on the others, too.

That's why it's possible for us to create an action plan to help tackle not just your PCOS symptoms but also the long-term health risks associated with them with one basic approach. And the best thing about it is that you're the one in control, supported by your healthcare professionals.

It's not uncommon, when you first learn of the negative risks associated with having PCOS, to feel a sense of helplessness. How can you lose weight if the odds are stacked against you and you're also faced with the possibility of diabetes, cancer or heart disease? What chance have you got when your body produces too much insulin, slows down your metabolism and makes it hard to lose weight?

The important thing to realize is that you *do* have control over the major PCOS triggers and risk factors – what you eat, your weight and your lifestyle. There's a lot of really simple stuff you can do to help yourself dramatically.

'In recent years, increasing attention has been paid to aspects of PCOS other than those related to fertility, in particular the long-term health implications,' says PCOS expert Gabor Kovacs. Kovacs believes that insulin-sensitizing drugs, such as metformin, show great promise – but he also acknowledges the importance of self-care, 'recommendations of mild to moderate exercise, dietary changes as well as taking part in programmes such as those aimed at stopping smoking, remain the best preventative health measures we can offer patients at the present moment.' And these are all preventative steps you can take yourself.

THE 80/20 RULE

Changing the way you eat, taking time out to relax and building exercise into your routine when you may feel tired or self-conscious is going to be a slow process. And you can't just try on these changes for a few weeks and then go back to your old habits. Eating right and living well are long-term goals to help you live the rest of your life feeling the best that you can.

The changes outlined in this Protection Plan are aimed at getting right to the heart of the problems that cause PCOS and increase the risk of long-term health complications – but getting to the heart of any problem takes time, patience and effort. Be realistic about making these changes. There's no point setting yourself impossible goals; you'll just make yourself feel like a failure when you don't reach them. While the plan advises healthy living, don't beat yourself up if you can't stick to it 100 per cent of the time and simply can't resist a chocolate bar or a greasy burger and fries or a day off exercise. See it as a special occasion, enjoy it and move on – and remind yourself of the 80/20 rule. As long as you try to get it right 80 per cent of the time, you can afford a day off now and again.

Commitment without pain

To stay focused and on track with the Protection Plan, try making some promises to yourself to help you stay committed:

I promise to:

- eat healthy, nutritious and delicious food because it gives me energy and fights PCOS
- exercise because it makes me feel good
- continue to learn about PCOS
- talk to my doctor about PCOS
- join a PCOS support group
- never beat myself up if I gain a pound or miss a workout. I will try harder tomorrow
- control my diet instead of letting my diet control me
- stay upbeat and not let my symptoms define how I feel
- see each day as a new beginning

It can be hard, but also you should try not feel persecuted because you have PCOS. Making healthy lifestyle changes are basic ways to feel healthier and live longer whether you have PCOS or not. It's just that these changes will make more of a difference because you happen to have PCOS.

STAYING MOTIVATED

The Protection Plan is designed to help you implement practical changes in your day-to-day life that will make a difference to the way you feel now and help prevent long-term threats to your health. For ease of reference we've summarized the information into two sections: Diet and Lifestyle. It typically takes two to three months on the Protection Plan to start to feel the health benefits and to see a reduction in your symptoms, although even after a week or two most women will notice considerable improvements. 'In general about four to six weeks is a crucial turning-point on any healthy eating programme,' says Nutritionist Dr Ann Walker from the University of Reading. 'Around that time, blood sugar levels start to stabilize and you should see a reduction in symptoms and an improvement in the way you feel.'

For example, the Hearts for Life programme in the US is designed to identify risk factors for heart disease and educate people about how to reduce them, but benefits aren't typically seen until the three-month stage.[1] Other research, this time on people with diabetes, shows improvements in cholesterol levels after three months of diet and lifestyle changes.[2] Another study, led by Professor John Holloszy from Washington University School of Medicine in St Louis, and reported in the April 2004 proceedings of the National Academy of Sciences, examined a group of people, average age 50, who avoided processed foods and made other healthy changes to their diet. After six months they were found to have increased energy and a greater sense of well-being, and their levels of bad (LDL) cholesterol were exceptionally low. In addition, their blood pressure readings were similar to those of the average 10 year old!

In other words, while this isn't an overnight sensation or a 'miracle cure', eating right for PCOS and taking good care of yourself will bring you amazing benefits if you're patient and stick with it.

A really good way to be able to reflect on how things are changing for you is to sit and write a list of the things that you're worried about now and want to change. For example, low energy levels that mean you don't have as much fun with your kids as you want to, crankiness when you're hungry that makes you snap at your partner when you get in from work, overweight that leaves you out of breath climbing the stairs, high cholesterol or high blood pressure that put your health at risk, insulin resistance that your doctor is concerned about. Write your list and give every item on it a rating from 1 to 100 to reflect how serious you feel it is before you start the plan. Then, tell your doctor, family and friends who will support you that you're starting the plan, and every four weeks, sit down and revisit this – and rate each item again. This way, you'll be able to see what progress you're making. Also, ask your doctor to measure your cholesterol, blood pressure and insulin resistance after you have been using the Protection Plan for three months. It's a real boost when you start to notice those little differences that make a big impact on your quality of life.

Your doctor and your plan

There's no doubt that medication can play an important role in controlling the symptoms of PCOS. You should keep in close contact with your doctor to assess your risk and discuss your options. (In fact, whenever you start a new diet and exercise routine it's important to discuss it with your doctor – especially if you're overweight.) However, whether or not you're on medication, PCOS is a lifelong condition that responds better when you take charge and start to manage it yourself.

START RIGHT NOW

When's the best time to start the Protection Plan? The answer is simple: now. You can let PCOS control your health and well-being or you can learn to take control. Don't let PCOS decide how much you get out of life. Find the motivation, the commitment and the time to put your health first. Start making positive changes today.

REFERENCES

1. Kirk Gardener, R. *et al.*, 'Hearts for Life: a community program on heart health promotion', *Can J Cardiovasc Nurs* 2003; 13 (1): 5–10
2. Kaplan, M. R. *et al.*, 'Prospective evaluation of HDL cholesterol changes after diet and physical conditioning programs for patients with type II diabetes mellitus', *Diabetes Care* 1985 Jul-Aug; 8 (4): 343–8

10 Protection on a Plate

66 *Once I started to understand the connection between the food I was eating and my symptoms, I started to feel much better. I stopped feeling tired all the time and woke up eager to start the day instead of wishing it was over all. Best of all, I got my waistline back.* 99

Ann, 39

66 *It's simple really. Eat better and you can change your life for the better. It took being diagnosed with PCOS for me to fully appreciate the huge impact food has on my health, my mood, my weight and my symptoms. I've learned the hard way that you really are what you eat.* 99

Shane, 31

It's clear that a poor diet can trigger or make the symptoms of PCOS worse. Healthy eating is a crucial step on your journey back to better health – now and in the future.

The food you eat plays a key role when it comes to hormonal balance – and that means all your hormones, including insulin and the stress hormone cortisol. All these hormones are linked together by your body's endocrine system. So what affects one has a knock-on effect on them all.

If you've got PCOS, not only do you metabolize food more slowly than a woman without PCOS, but high blood sugar levels and insulin resistance cause your body to react in the opposite way to what you really want – you store more energy as fat rather than burning it off. And as we've seen, high blood sugar, insulin resistance and overweight all put your long-term health at risk.

What's more, high levels of insulin and excess body fat also trigger an increase in androgens and oestrogens. Many of the frustrating symptoms of PCOS, such as irregular periods, excess hair growth and acne, are caused by excessive production of these sex hormones.

So what's the most effective way to fight back against all this? If you make sure your body isn't set up to stimulate insulin and androgen production in the first place, you can really help to reduce your symptoms now and any health risks later on. The best way to do that is to eat foods that can help keep blood sugar levels stable and that don't trigger an insulin response.

PCOS-FRIENDLY DIET GUIDELINES

A well-balanced, nutritious, whole-food, low-glycaemic index (GI), ideally organic diet can have a positive effect on women with PCOS, easing their symptoms and reducing the long-term health risks. It may at first be tough to make all the changes we recommend, so don't try and make them all at once. Every small change will make a difference, and encourage you to make the next one. From our experience, and from talking to other women with PCOS who have changed their diet and lifestyle – often with dramatic results – the order in which we have listed these changes makes for the easiest way to start putting them into action. Try each change and stick to it until you feel comfortable about moving on to the next one – this could be a couple of days or a couple of weeks; just take it at your own pace.

A WHOLEFOOD DIET

Eat as many fresh and delicious wholefoods as you can. Wholefoods are foods in their most natural form, like fresh fruits, vegetables, wholegrains, fish, nuts and seeds. They've had no nutrients or fibre taken away, and no colourings, flavourings or preservatives added. Your body loves wholefoods because it can process and digest them really easily, getting access to all their goodness without having to work extra hard to get rid of any junk at the same time. Wholefoods that are produced organically, without the use of potentially dangerous chemicals and pesticides, are even better for you because they contain fewer chemicals for your body to process.

As well as nutrients, the fibre in wholefoods is particularly beneficial for women with PCOS.[1] Fibre can reduce oestrogen levels by preventing excess oestrogen from being reabsorbed into the blood. Fresh fruits and vegetables, legumes (peas and beans) seeds, nuts and grains are excellent sources of fibre – eat them as snacks, salads, sandwich fillings, bakes, and in smoothies, soups and casseroles.

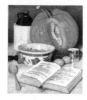

SAMPLE MENU

A good day's menu high in wholefoods could be:

- *Breakfast:* Muesli with chopped fruit
- *Mid-morning:* A smoothie (whiz up a banana, a handful of raspberries, strawberries or half a mango and a splash of soya milk in a blender)
- *Lunch:* Lean fish, chicken or hummus sandwich with onion and tomato on wholegrain bread, with a side salad plus an apple and some almonds
- *Mid-afternoon:* A peach and a low-fat yoghurt
- *Dinner:* A three-bean chilli with wholegrain rice, a green salad and a bowl of cherries or chopped pineapple for dessert.

There are more menu ideas on page 77, and the Recipes chapter will also help you make wholefoods part of your everyday diet.

LESS SUGAR, FEWER REFINED CARBS

Once you've got into the swing of eating more wholefoods, it's time to cut down on refined carbohydrates (which your body turns into sugar very fast) and sugar itself. Sugar consumption has been linked with many disorders, from diabetes to heart disease and cancer.[2] If that weren't enough, sugar contains nothing but empty calories and goes right to your bloodstream, where it raises blood sugar, triggers the release of insulin, aggravates your PCOS symptoms, makes you gain weight and increases your long-term health risks.

If you need another reason to lay off the sugar, research also shows that sugar reduces the ability of white blood cells to fight infection, making you more prone to colds and illness.

But before you start to panic about giving up everything sweet, don't forget that your body can get all the sugar and energy it needs from natural sources like fruits and unrefined carbohydrates such as grains and lentils. And with the 80/20 rule (eat healthy foods 80 per cent of the time and you can afford the occasional indulgence), you can treat yourself to something sweet from time to time – a dark chocolate bar, a fruity yoghurt, a piece of fruit tart or a wholewheat blueberry muffin are all great choices. Even the occasional blowout on cream cakes or other sugar-laden morsels won't kill you as long as you get back on track the next day.

We're not saying you can't ever eat anything sweet again – but you need to cut out sugar and refined carbs most of the time to give your body the protection it needs from daily PCOS symptoms and the threat of diabetes. And though it may seem hard to believe when you first start out, after a while you'll find your body loses its taste for sugar and you won't be hankering after it anymore.

Tips for avoiding sugar

Cut out processed foods
The US Department of Agriculture estimates that the average American consumes at least 64 pounds of sugar a year; the UK is close behind. Most of this sugar doesn't come from the sugar bowl on the table but is hidden in our foods – not just in cakes, sweets and pastries but in juices and refined, processed, pre-packaged foods. So get into the habit

of reading food labels to avoid those hidden sugars. Check the labels of your favourite sauces, spreads, cereals, biscuits, cakes and bread — you may be surprised at the amount of sugar lurking there, under one of its many aliases: dextrose, glucose, sucrose, fructose, lactose, maltose, corn syrup, cane sugar, muscovado sugar, honey, treacle, syrup, molasses, etc.

Also, limit your intake of sweets, biscuits, cakes, pies, doughnuts, pastries and other sweet baked foods or processed refined foods with sugar added in. Eat fresh fruit instead or choose muffins, dried fruit or wholemeal scones. Look for breakfast cereals that contain no more than 5 grams of sugar per serving. The best bets are wholegrain cereals like muesli, granola, wheat flakes or hot oat or wheat cereals.

Go for brown, not white!
Brown rice, pasta and bread are made from wholegrains — and include fibre to help slow down your body's conversion of carbohydrates into blood sugar (glucose). This means you get a steady release of sugar into your bloodstream and you'll avoid the highs and lows that can lead to mood swings and the cravings for sugary foods that just make the problems like insulin resistance and weight gain worse.

Don't be fooled by 'fat-free'
Bear in mind that fat-free foods often replace fat with sugar, which makes them worse than their fatty counterparts for women with PCOS.

Mind what you drink
Fruit drinks, beverages and cocktails are essentially sugar loaded non-carbonated soda pop. Most popular brands contain only 5 to 10 per cent juice. If you do choose them, go for high-juice brands and water them down with spring water, or choose freshly pressed juice and add water to it.

Avoid sugar substitutes
Sugar substitutes aren't a good idea if you've got PCOS. Many metabolically challenged people find these cause problems like headaches and

stomach upsets.[3] Honey and maple syrup may sound healthier, but unfortunately they aren't. A tiny pinch of sugar is OK if you really need some sweetness but better to add natural sweeteners like fruit juice or fresh fruit, or try the herbal alternative Stevia, available at health food stores, which is sweet tasting and has no calories.

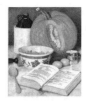

SAMPLE MENU

A great low-sugar menu would be the same as the wholefood menu above, or try these suggestions (for more ideas see our the Recipes chapter):

- *Breakfast:* I boiled egg with wholegrain toast and a pear
- *Mid-morning:* I apple with a handful of cashews
- *Lunch:* a big Greek salad with red onions, feta cheese, juicy tomatoes, olives and cucumber sprinkled with mixed seeds, with wholemeal pitta bread plus a slice of watermelon
- *Mid-afternoon:* 2 wholegrain crackers with cottage cheese and a sprinkling of sesame seeds
- *Dinner:* Chicken strips or tofu stir fry with crunchy mange-tout, broccoli, carrots, peppers, beansprouts and onions, and a sliced mango for dessert.

Make the GI work for you

Once you're eating more delicious fresh wholefoods, and less sugar, it's time to get to grips with low-glycaemic index (GI) foods to get your blood sugar into even better shape and help reduce insulin resistance. This will boost your protection from diabetes and weight gain even more, as well as helping to keep your PCOS symptoms under control.

The glycaemic index was designed for use by people with diabetes. It ranks food by the influence they have on your blood sugar level a few hours after you eat them. Pure glucose is used as the reference food, and its index value is set at 100. All other foods are then compared to glucose and ranked accordingly.

Foods with a GI of 70 or more are called high-glycaemic index foods as they trigger a rapid increase in blood sugar; foods with a GI of 55–69 are called medium-glycaemic index foods as they trigger a medium increase; foods with a GI below 55 are called low-glycaemic foods because they have only a moderate to low impact on blood sugar. For example, mashed potatoes (GI = 70) are classified as 'high glycaemic' because when you eat them your body turns the carbs they contain into blood sugar very quickly. By contrast, lentils (GI = 29) are a low-glycaemic food because it takes your body a lot longer to digest them and release their sugar into your blood.

As a rough guide you're generally better off eating complex carbo-hydrates (vegetables, wholegrains, legumes) instead of simple ones (cakes, sweets, sugar) because complex carbohydrates take longer to digest and absorb, and usually have a less dramatic impact on your blood sugar levels than simple sugars. That's the basic rule for PCOS.

'A low-GI diet is a sensible option for women with PCOS,' says PCOS expert Adam Balen, 'if you're insulin resistant it makes sense to steer away from foods with a high glycaemic rating, as these kinds of foods trigger an increase in blood sugar and a greater insulin response.' Numerous studies have found that eating foods low on the glycaemic index improves glucose tolerance and insulin function and therefore reduces the risk of obesity, diabetes, syndrome X and heart disease.[4]

As a rule, refined or processed foods generally have a higher glycaemic index. For example, the glycaemic index for rice cakes is 78, vs 55 for brown rice. Corn flakes are high, at 81 vs sweet corn at 54. The less refined or processed a food is, the lower its glycaemic index will be. So eating foods in their natural form – or as wholefoods – is very much to your advantage.

Now, we've said you should be choosing *wholefoods* that are low on the GI index, not just low-GI foods full stop. This is an important point for women with PCOS. GI alone is not a great way to determine how PCOS-friendly a food is. You'll see from the chart on pages 81–83 that, for example, ice cream and sponge cake are relatively low on the GI scale, because they're high in fat, and fat slows down the speed at which your body releases sugar from a meal. But if you have PCOS, you need to avoid foods like these as well.

Equally, you'll see that some really nutritious foods like broad beans, parsnips and pineapples are high on the GI list, because your body can break them down to release their sugars quickly. But you'd be better choosing a dessert of pineapple than a bar of chocolate because the pineapple will also give you lots of vitamins, minerals and fibre instead of fat, sugar and empty calories.

So how can you make the most of the GI index to reduce PCOS symptoms now and protect yourself from diabetes in the future? The answer is to make the GI index work for you.

For example, you can make useful food substitutions that will lower the glycaemic index of a snack or a meal. Some people consider a bran muffin (GI = 60) a healthy snack. But actually, a small apple (GI = 37) is a much better choice. Or, if you're having carbs as part of a main meal, sweet potatoes (GI = 54) are a better choice than mashed white potatoes (GI = 70).

You can also note if a nutritious food like pineapple or broad beans is surprisingly high on the GI list – and reduce its impact on your blood sugar by combining it with a protein or high-fibre food to slow down the speed at which your body can process it. Both fibre and protein act to slow down your body's digestion, and can be mixed with healthy but high-GI foods to reduce their impact on your blood sugar (and therefore your insulin) levels.

For example, have a bran muffin with low-fat cottage cheese, a slice of rye bread with hummus, a baked potato with low-fat cheddar and a big green salad, or pea soup with a generous sprinkling of seeds and a wholegrain pitta stuffed with lean chicken. This way, you'll benefit from all the essential vitamins and minerals in a high-GI food while minimizing its effect on your blood sugar.

You also need to consider that although some foods don't rank high on the glycaemic index, they are carbohydrate dense – that is, they contain a lot of carbs for the amount of bulk they provide. Examples would include whole grains, some legumes such as pinto beans or tinned kidney beans, and starchy vegetables such as potatoes. The total amount of insulin your body produces depends not only on a food's GI rating, but also its carbohydrate density (also known as its glycaemic load (GL) – see box on pages 84–5) – because the more carbohydrate you eat, the more insulin you produce. So while some legumes, for example, don't cause a quick high rise in blood sugar, they can promote a longer, lower rise which needs to be monitored closely.

In other words, while the GI index is a brilliant source of information about food and how it affects your blood sugar, it isn't a foolproof way to create a healthy diet to fight your PCOS symptoms or protect your long-term health. You have to keep an eye on carb content and portion size (the *glycaemic load*) to make the best PCOS-friendly food choices.

Low-GI foods for PCOS

- Vegetables like broccoli, lettuce, celery, cabbage, cucumber, parsley, radishes, spinach, turnips and watercress. They're packed with nutrients and have four to ten times less carbohydrate than other vegetables.
- Less carbohydrate-dense legumes such as fresh-cooked kidney beans, soy beans, lentils, black-eyed peas, chickpeas and lima beans that induce low blood sugar and insulin response (better than tinned kidney beans, pinto beans, navy beans or peas).
- Low-carbohydrate fruits such as strawberries, raspberries, grapefruit, apples, cherries, peaches, pears and plums.

Table 1 A to Z of GI foods

Food item	Glycaemic index	Food item	Glycaemic index
BEANS, LEGUMES AND NUTS		Bran muffin, 80g	60
Baked beans, tinned, 120g	48	Bun, hamburger, 50g	61
Black beans, 120g	30	Croissant, 1	67
Black-eyed beans, 120g	42	Crumpet, 50g	69
Broad beans, 80g	79	Dark rye, 1 slice	76
Butter beans, 70g	31	Doughnut, 40g	76
Chick peas, boiled 120g	33	Flan cake, 1 slice	65
Haricot beans, 90g	38	French baguette, 30g	95
Kidney beans, 90g	27	Fruit loaf, 1 slice	47
Kidney beans, tinned, 95g	52	Gluten-free bread, 1 slice	90
Lentils, 95g	29	Light rye, 1 slice	55
Peanuts, roasted, salted, 75g	14	Linseed rye, 1 slice	55
Peas, dried, 70g	22	Melba toast, 4 squares	70
Peas, green, fresh, frozen,		Pastry, flaky, 65g	59
boiled, 80g	48	Pumpernickel, 2 slices	41
Pinto beans, tinned 95g	45	Pitta bread, 1 piece	57
Soya beans, boiled, 90g	18	Pitta bread, 65g	57
Split peas, yellow, boiled, 90g	32	Pizza, cheese and tomato, 2 slices	60
		Pound cake, 1 slice, 80g	54
BISCUITS		Rye bread, 1 slice	65
Digestives plain, 2	59	Sourdough rye, 1 slice	65
Milk arrowroot, 2	63	Sponge cake, 1 slice	46
Morning coffee, 3	79	Taco shells, 26g	68
Oatmeal, 3	54	White, 1 slice	70
Rich tea, 2	55	Wholemeal, 1 slice	69
Shortbread, 2	64		
Vanilla wafers, 6	77	**BREAKFAST CEREALS**	
Wheatmeal, 2	62	All-bran, 40g	42
		Bran Buds, 30g	58
BRAN		Cheerios, 30g	74
Oat bran, 10g	55	Coco Pops, 30g	77
Rice bran, 10g	19	Cornflakes, 30g	81
		Muesli, 60g	43
BREADS AND CAKES		Oat bran, 10g	55
Apple muffin, 1	44	Porridge, 245g	42
Angel food cake, 30g	67	Rice Bran, 10g	19
Bagel, 1 white	72	Rice Krispies, 30g	82
Banana cake, 1 slice	47	Shredded Wheat, 25g	67
Blackbread, dark rye, 1 slice	76		
Blueberry muffin	59		

continued

Table 1 A to Z of GI foods (*continued*)

Food item	Glycaemic index	Food item	Glycaemic index
Special K, 30g	54	Cherries, 80g	22
Sultana Bran, 45g	52	Fruit cocktail, 125g	55
Weetabix, 2	69	Grapefruit juice, 250ml	48
		Grapefruit, raw, 100g	25
CRACKERS		Grapes, green, 100g	46
Crispbread, 20g	81	Kiwifruit, 80g	52
Rice cakes, 2	82	Lychee, 90g	79
Ryvita, 20g	69	Mango, 1 small	55
Waterbiscuits, 20g	78	Orange, 1 medium	44
		Orange juice, 250ml	46
DAIRY PRODUCTS		Peach, 1 large	42
Custard, 175g	43	Peach, tinned, heavy syrup, 125g	58
Ice cream, full fat, 2 scoops	61	Pear, 1 medium	38
Ice cream, low fat, 2 scoops	50	Pears, tinned in juice, 125g	44
Milk, chocolate, 30g	49	Pineapple, fresh, 2 slices	66
Milk, full fat, 250ml	27	Pineapple juice, 250g	46
Milk, skimmed, 250ml	32	Plums 3–4, small	39
Tapioca pudding, 250g	81	Raisins, 40g	64
Yogurt, low-fat, fruit, 200g	33	Sultanas, 40g	56
Yogurt, low-fat artificial		Watermelon, 150g	72
sweetener, 200g	14		
		GRAINS, RICE AND PASTA	
DRINKS		Basmati white rice, boiled, 180g	25
Cola, 1 can	63	Buckwheat, 80g	54
Orange squash, 250ml	66	Capellini pasta, 180g	45
		Cornmeal, 40g	68
FISH, PORK, SOYA		Couscous,120g	65
Fish fingers, 125g	38	Fettucini, 180g	32
Sausages, fried, 2	28	Glutinous rice, white, 174g	98
Tofu, 100g	100	Gnocchi, 145g	68
		Linguini pasta, 180g	55
FRUITS AND FRUIT JUICES		Macaroni, cooked, 190g	45
Apple, 1 small	38	Noodles, 85g packet, cooked	46
Apple, 1 medium	67	Ravioli, meat-filled, cooked, 20g	39
Apple juice, fresh pressed		Rice cakes	78
unsweetened, 250ml	40	Rice, instant, cooked, 180g	87
Apricots, 3 medium	57	Rice, brown	55
Apricots, tinned, 125g	64	Semolina, 230g	55
Apricots, dried, 30g	31	Spaghetti, white, cooked, 180g	37
Banana, 1 medium	55		
Breadfruit, 120g	68		

continued

Table 1 A to Z of GI foods (*continued*)

Food item	Glycaemic index	Food item	Glycaemic index
Spaghetti, wholemeal, cooked, 180g	37	Mars bar, 60g	68
		Popcorn, 20g	55
SOUPS		Potato crisps, plain, 50g	54
Black bean soup, 220ml	64	Pretzels, 50g	83
Green pea soup, tinned, 220ml	66		
Lentil soup, tinned, 220ml	44	VEGETABLES	
Pea and ham soup, 220ml	60	Beetroot, 2–3 slices	64
Split pea soup, 220ml	60	Carrots, 70g	49
Tomato soup, 220ml	38	Maize, 40g	68
		Parsnips, 75g	97
SUGARS		Potato, baked, 1 medium	85
Fructose, 10g	23	Potato, new, boiled, 175g	62
Glucose	100	Potatoes, French fried, 120g	75
Honey, 20g	58	Potatoes, mashed, 120g	70
Maltose, pure, 10g	100	Sweet corn, 85g	55
Sucrose, 1 teaspoon	65	Sweet potato, 80g	54
		Swede, 60g	72
SWEETS AND SNACKS			
Jelly beans, 10g	80		

Just as a low- or no-carbohydrate diet isn't a cure for PCOS, as you miss out on good-quality protein and the energy boost that carbohydrates can give you, a low-GI diet isn't a cure-all, either. Some foods with relatively high glycaemic ratings, such as broad beans, brown rice or dried fruit, provide important nutrients. And eating lots of cheese and ice cream because they have a relatively low GI isn't a good idea, as they're high in calories so can make you put on weight. Try to use the GI as a useful source of information, not a foolproof guide to PCOS diet rules.

The glycaemic load

Once you've got the hang of GI, you can refine your food choices even further by choosing foods according to their glycaemic *load* as well.

The GI has given us part of the story – it's taught us that indeed not all carbohydrates are created equal, based on eating 50 grams of carbs per food listed, but the GI alone also makes it very difficult for folks like you and me to look at a plate full of food and calculate if the combined meal is actually high, moderate or low GI. What the GL does is help you work out how much of an effect on your blood sugar the average portion size of a food will have – whether it is low or high GI. This measure is the glycaemic load, which can be calculated by multiplying the carbohydrate content per serving by the food's glycaemic index number. So if the GI of a food is 71, treat this as 71% when you multiply it by the grams of carbohydrate in a serving.

Here's an example of the perspective you get by calculating glycaemic load. Judging from their high glycaemic index – up to 97 in some studies – carrots would seem to be a food to avoid if you are carbohydrate-sensitive. But to get 50 grams of carbohydrates from carrots, you would have to eat a lot of them because the percentage of carbohydrate is low. A half-cup serving of carrots contains only 6.2 grams of carbs, so the glycaemic load of that portion would be 6.2 × 97%, or 6, a low value. By contrast, a plain five-ounce bagel provides 65 grams of carbohydrate and has a GI of 72. Its glycaemic load (65 × 72%) is a whopping 47.

Foods with a low glycaemic load rank from one to 10; those with medium load range from 11–19 and those with high glycaemic load rank at 20 or above. You can find examples of glycaemic load rankings of various foods at http://www.mendosa.com/gilists.htm and www.50plus.org/Libraryitems/2_5_glycemicload.html.

So, what all this information on GI and GL tells you, in the end, is that wholefoods are generally a good bet, portion control is important, and if you think a food's high GI, then eat some protein or fibre with it. What we're saying is, use GI and GL info to help you work out the best PCOS-friendly foods, but don't get carried away doing calculations for everything you eat. As we've always stressed moderation is everything and you can always make better choices about carbohydrates simply by replacing processed and refined foods (such as snack foods, white bread and sugary desserts) with fruits, starchy vegetables (such as sweet potatoes and winter squash), whole grains and beans.

LESS SALT

Once your health-protection diet is well under way, and you've a solid understanding of the benefits of wholefoods, less sugar and the GI rating of different foods, you need to consider protecting yourself against high blood pressure and bloating.[5] Cutting down on salt is a great way to do this.

You might be thinking, 'But I never add salt to my food.' That's a great start. But salt is often used as a preservative and is added to most processed, pre-packaged foods before you even put them on the table. If you eat a lot of processed foods, you're taking in more hidden salt than you realize. And if you add salt when you cook, that counts, too. It goes without saying that if you add salt at the table or to your cooking, cut back right now.

You'll gradually find that when you start cutting back on salt you do adjust and learn to appreciate the more subtle flavours that were once hidden by the over-powering taste of salt.

Here are some easy ways to protect yourself from hidden salt in your food:

Gradually wean yourself from salty foods and the habit of adding salt automatically to food and to your cooking. Instead of salt, experiment with lemon juice, wine, mustard or vinegar. Better still, try herbs and spices to flavour your food. Basil, dill, fennel and garlic work well with salads. Thyme, tarragon and parsley can really enhance the flavour of meat, fish and vegetables. In addition to their role as flavour-enhancers, herbs and spices can be particularly useful for PCOS sufferers, as many have protective health benefits (see below). If you find that low-fat or low-salt foods taste bland, you can use herbs to enhance the flavour of virtually any dish, including desserts. Generally, herbs are delicately flavoured, so add them to your cooking in the last few minutes. It helps to taste-test, too. Too few herbs will contribute nothing to your dish, while too many will overpower the other ingredients.

Try:

- Basil – for pesto, tomato sauce, tomato soup, tomato juice, potato dishes, prawns, meat, chicken and poultry, pasta, rice and egg dishes
- Bay leaves – for soups, stews, casseroles, meat and poultry marinades, stocks
- Chilli – for meat, chicken and poultry, prawns, shellfish and tomato dishes, curries
- Chives – for salads, chicken, soups, cheese dishes, egg dishes, mayonnaise, vinaigrettes
- Coriander – for stir fries, curries, soups, salads, with seafood
- Dill – for salads, sauces, fish, sour cream, cheese and potato dishes
- Fennel – for stuffings, sauces, seafood
- Garlic – for soups, sauces, pasta, meat, chicken, shellfish, pesto, salad dressings and bread
- Ginger – for cakes, biscuits, curries or Chinese-style dishes
- Lemongrass – for Thai, Indian or Chinese dishes, stir fries, curries, seafood, soups, or as a tea
- Marjoram – for meat, fish, egg dishes, cheese dishes, pizza
- Mint – for drinks, confectionery, meat, chicken, yoghurt, desserts, sauces, vegetable dishes
- Oregano – for cheese dishes, egg dishes, tomato sauce, pizza, meat, stuffing, bread, pasta
- Parsley – for pesto, egg dishes, pasta, rice dishes, salads, butter, sauces, seafood, vegetable dishes
- Rosemary – for fish, poultry, meat, bread, sauces, soups

- Sage – for stuffings, tomato dishes, cheese dishes
- Tarragon – for salad dressing, egg dishes
- Thyme – for chowders, bread, chicken and poultry, soups, stock, stews, stuffings, with butter, cheese, mayonnaise, mustard, vinegar.

Smoked and pickled foods

Also, avoid foods such as cured and smoked meats, smoked and pickled fish, tinned meats, salted butters/margarines, salted nuts, biscuits, beans and vegetables in brine, olives in brine, sauces, ketchup, stock cubes and tinned fish in brine. (Oily fish and bread are highly salted foods but they shouldn't be avoided as they provide other important and protective nutrients.) Go instead for the low-salt alternatives such as fresh fish, fresh lean meats, unsalted butter, nuts, dried fruits, beans and vegetables tinned with no added salt, olives in oil, and low-salt versions of sauces, stock cubes and ketchup.

Become a sodium sleuth

Many foods today claim to be reduced salt or low salt, but this can be confusing when the labels talk of sodium. To find out how much salt is in a food, multiply the sodium content on the label by 2.5. You should aim for less than 5g of salt a day.

Calcium boost for blood pressure

As well as cutting down on salt, you can help reduce your risk of high blood pressure by making sure you get enough calcium. Good sources are low-fat dairy products, leafy green vegetables including spinach and cabbage, sesame seeds, nuts such as almonds, and tofu.

SAMPLE MENU

A great low-salt menu for the day could be similar to the low-sugar or high-wholefoods menus suggested above, or you could try these alternatives:

- *Breakfast:* Porridge with chopped banana and sesame seeds
- *Mid-morning:* 2 plums and a handful of almonds
- *Lunch:* Grilled salmon steak or tofu patty with steamed green vegetables and a baked sweet potato, plus a bowl of strawberries
- *Mid-afternoon:* 2 rice cakes with cottage cheese
- *Dinner:* Roasted Mediterranean vegetables (peppers, courgettes, onions, tomatoes) with chickpeas, basil and chives; plus a soya yoghurt.

THE RIGHT FATS

The next part of your PCOS-fighting diet is all about the fats you eat.

The first thing to get to grips with is that you need to avoid saturated fats. Found in dairy produce and meat, these animal fats contain unhealthy kinds of prostaglandins that encourage blood-clotting and inflammation, as well as hormones and antibiotics that can upset your hormonal, immune and digestive systems. What's more, saturated fats contribute to weight gain, block other nutrients, interfere with the absorption of EFAs (essential fatty acids – see page 89) and stimulate oestrogen production.

Vegetable oils in the form of fried, oxidized or hydrogenated fats, as found in margarine, vegetable shortenings, many processed foods, snacks and fast foods, are also bad news. These transfatty acids should be avoided because they increase your risk of diabetes and heart disease, according to research reported in the *New England Journal of Medicine*.[6]

Also known as *hydrogenated* fats or oils, the risk they pose to heart health is considered so major that new manufacturing guidelines are being laid down by the US and UK governments to reduce the amount of transfats in foods. The US Dietary Guidelines Association recommends that transfats should be kept below 1 per cent of total daily calories.

Avoiding saturates

Choose low-fat dairy products and spreads, white meat, fish, and lean cuts of red meat. When you can, try to buy organic produce that's free of antibiotics, steroids and pesticides, too.

Avoiding transfats

This is harder in some ways – many margarines are full of them, but you can get some (such as Pure Organic in the UK) which have the qualities of a margarine without the transfats. Equally, it might be worth thinking about using a small amount of butter or a spreadable butter that has some olive oil added, rather than eating margarine.

Good fats

But you shouldn't be avoiding fat altogether – a diet that protects you from diabetes, heart disease and PCOS symptoms is one that supplies you with good fats, or EFAs (essential fatty acids), as they're massively beneficial to your health (they're not called 'essential' fats for nothing!).[7] Aim for a diet that's 50 per cent carbohydrates (wholefood and low GI, of course!), 20 to 25 per cent good-quality protein, and about 20 to 25 per cent healthy fats.

Unsaturated fats (also called *polyunsaturated* or *monounsaturated* fats) have a protective effect on your heart. You'll find them in olive oil and foods such as avocados, but the real stars for women with PCOS are the Omega 3 oils (and, to a lesser extent, the Omega 6 oils). Both of these occur naturally in oily fish, nuts and seeds – and your body has to get them from your diet because it can't manufacture them itself. Every single cell in your body needs EFAs such as these to maintain a flexible cell wall that can take in nutrients and push out toxins. They're also important for hormonal balance, as your body needs them to produce ovarian and stress hormones. As for heart protection, they help your body to make the healthy kind of prostaglandins (hormone-like substances which, among other benefits, help to reduce abnormal blood clotting).

Finally, a lack of EFAs can make PCOS symptoms worse and actually increase your risk of insulin resistance and weight gain. This is because EFAs slow down the passage of carbohydrates into your system, thus keeping blood sugar and insulin levels lower and your PCOS symptoms at bay. EFAs are, in fact, one of the best blood-sugar stabilizers – and stable blood sugar means a reduction in symptoms and less likelihood of insulin resistance, diabetes, heart disease, stroke, obesity and depression.

In other words, a low-fat diet is *not* the right diet for fighting PCOS. You need fats – but, as with carbohydrates, you need to choose the right kind.[8]

Action plan for including more EFAs in your diet

So, we know that Omega 6 and Omega 3 are the best fats for PCOS. Omega 6 fats are much more common in Western diets, found in foods such as leafy green vegetables and sunflower, soy, olive, sesame, coconut and peanut oils. Omega 3 fats are less common, present in the oils of cold water fish as well as in hemp and pumpkin seeds and in walnuts. You need to concentrate on getting a balance of both.

COOKING OILS

Popular oils such as olive, sunflower, sesame and corn, while containing varying amounts of Omega 6 contain negligible amounts of Omega 3. Of the readily available vegetable oils, only three contain both Omega 3 and Omega 6: flaxseed, hempseed and soy oil.

SOMETHING FISHY

Oily fish (mackerel, salmon, herrings and sardines) are rich in Omega 3 EFAs. Aim to eat oily fish at least twice a week, but no more than three or four times a week. If you don't eat fish, you can try sea vegetables (seaweeds), used in Japanese cooking in dishes such as sushi and soups.

SOWING THE SEEDS

Flaxseed oil or flax seeds — also known as linseed — are also a great source of Omega 3. Try a daily dose of 3 teaspoons of cold-pressed flaxseed oil or three tablespoons of ground flax seed. You can also use the oil or seeds in salad dressings and smoothies.

Use only cold-pressed vegetable oils; the bottle should say 'unrefined' or 'unhydrated' as well as 'cold-pressed'. You may also like to grind some seeds and mix them into cereal or sprinkle them over salads.

Seeds such as sunflower, pumpkin, hemp and sesame, and nuts such as almonds, cashews and walnuts are all great sources of EFAs, so eat some every day, maybe as a snack between meals, or in flapjacks, on cereals or as a topping for salads and soups.

GET FRESH

Eating as much fresh wholefood as possible and avoiding refined and processed foods is also another way to help your body get the essential fatty acids it needs — because highly processed foods actually block the absorption of EFAs.

EFAs and weight loss

Some experts think that, as essential fats are needed in every cell membrane and by so many bodily processes, unlike the non-essential, saturated fats they don't travel to fat cells in your bum and thighs, but instead end up in the fabric of your body's cells.

SAMPLE MENU

For a great EFA-boosting menu for the day, try this:

- *Breakfast:* Luxury muesli made with cashews, almonds, sesame, flax seeds and chopped apple and soya milk
- *Mid-morning:* 1 peach and 5 walnuts
- *Lunch:* Barbecued sardines or tofu patty with a big green salad dressed with hemp oil, lemon juice and vinegar, plus a bowl of mixed fruit salad
- *Mid-afternoon:* A handful of Japanese rice crackers with seaweed and mixed seeds
- *Dinner:* Chunky vegetable soup with a multi-seed bagel or multi-seed bread, oat and seed flapjack slice with a pear.

REFERENCES

1. Biesalski, H. K. *et al.*, 'Diabetes preventive components in the Mediterranean diet', *Eur J Nutr* 2004 Mar; 43 Suppl 1: I26–I30; Rose, D. P. *et al.*, 'Effects of diet supplementation with wheat bran on serum estrogen levels in the follicular and luteal phases of the menstrual cycle', *Nutrition* 1997 Jun; 13 (6): 535–9

2. Bosseley, S. *et al.*, 'Political context of the World Health Organization: sugar industry threatens to scupper the WHO', *Int J Health Serv* 2003; 33 (4): 831–3

3. American Dietetic Association, 'Position of the American Dietetic Association: use of nutritive and non-nutritive sweeteners', *J Am Diet Assoc* 2004 Feb; 104 (2): 255–75

4. Bell, S. J. *et al.*, 'Low-glycemic-load diets: impact on obesity and chronic diseases', *Crit Rev Food Sci Nutr* 2003; 43 (4): 357–77

5. Srinath, R. K. *et al.*, 'Diet, nutrition and the prevention of hypertension and cardiovascular diseases', *Public Health Nutr* 2004 Feb; 7 (1A): 167–86

6. Hu, F. B. *et al.*, 'Dietary fat intake and the risk of coronary heart disease in women', *N Engl J Med* 1997 Nov 20; 337 (21): 1491–9

7. Lefevre, M. *et al.*, 'Dietary fatty acids, hemostasis, and cardiovascular disease risk', *J Am Diet Assoc* 2004 Mar; 104 (3): 410–19 (quiz page 492)

8. Kasim Karakas, M. C. *et al.*, 'Metabolic and endocrine effects of a polyunsaturated fatty acid-rich diet in polycystic ovary syndrome', *J Clin Endocrinol Metab* 2004 Feb; 89 (2): 615–20

11 Small Miracles: Water, Fibre and Other PCOS-friendly Nutrients

Once you're following the dietary guidelines recommended in the previous chapter, you'll be making a really positive contribution to keeping your PCOS under control and cutting your long-term health risks. Once you've got into the habit of eating in a PCOS-friendly way 80 per cent of the time, it's worth just fine-tuning by checking that you're getting enough of the following 'small miracle' foods into your diet, too.

WATER

Water is absolutely crucial if you've got PCOS. Your body is made up of two-thirds water, so water intake and distribution are vital for hormonal function. You need to drink a lot to keep your hormone system working at its best and to keep insulin resistance at bay. Water also helps your body metabolize stored fat by maximizing muscle function. It's therefore important in any healthy dietary programme.

Drinking enough water can also help reduce the risk of high blood pressure and heart disease. Recent research has shown that people who drink five or more 8-ounce glasses of water daily have significantly fewer heart attacks than those who drink two or fewer glasses a day.[1] It seems that dehydration increases the tendency for the blood to clot, whereas adequate hydration prevents excessive blood-clotting. Blood-clotting is a risk factor for heart disease. Seen in this light, drinking enough water isn't just a key requirement for nutrition and hormonal health: it could be a matter of life and death.

Action plan for drinking more water

On average you should aim to drink eight 8-ounce glasses of water a day.

If you don't think you're drinking enough, keep a record over the next few days. Any non-caffeinated fluids can be counted as fluid to meet your body's water needs. Caffeine raises sugar and insulin levels and acts as a diuretic, so caffeinated beverages such as tea, coffee and cola cannot be counted as fluids.

Are you drinking enough? If not, think of ways to include more fluids. Here are some ideas:

- If you get bored with drinking water all the time, try fresh fruit juice or diluted juice – but watch out for fruit juice drinks posing as fresh fruit juice; they're really just sugary, expensive fakes. Try some better quality squashes and cordials.
- Try herbal teas – they aren't, strictly speaking, teas, but just use that name as they are infused with hot water the way black teas are.
- Have a bottle of water handy when you're doing physical activity, watching TV, sitting at your desk or driving.
- Get into the habit of drinking a glass of water every time you brush your teeth or take your daily multivitamin and -mineral.
- Fill a pitcher or a bottle with your targeted amount and drink it throughout the day. If the container is empty by bedtime, you'll know you've achieved your goal.
- Don't forget that fruits and vegetables count towards your fluid intake because they consist of 90 per cent water. They also supply it in a form that's easy for your body to use, at the same time providing your body with a high percentage of vitamins and minerals.

ANTIOXIDANTS

You've probably heard of antioxidants; all the latest health and beauty products use them as their star ingredients to combat the signs of ageing and keep skin looking glowing and supple. You may also have read about how they help to prevent cancer and heart disease. All these reasons make antioxidants brilliant for women with PCOS.

Vitamins A, C and E are the most commonly mentioned antioxidants, but there are also many antioxidant compounds found in fruits, vegetables and sprouted grains. All of them promote good health in countless ways, and are particularly important for women with PCOS who are insulin resistant and at risk of developing diabetes and heart disease.[2]

Antioxidants work by combating a harmful chemical process known as *oxidation* that takes place in your body as part natural processes such as breathing, eating and exercising. Every chemical reaction in your body produces chemicals known as free radicals. Free radicals are unstable, highly reactive and potentially harmful molecules formed in the body and exacerbated by exposure to sunlight, cigarette smoke and environmental pollutants. Without intervention, free radicals wreak damage at a cellular level, accelerating the ageing process (wrinkles!) and compromising your immune system. In addition to diabetes, conditions as varied as cancer, heart disease, asthma, senility, arthritis and poor vision have all been linked to free-radical damage.

If you're eating a lot of fresh fruits and vegetables, as well as wholegrains and other fresh foods, your antioxidant intake is likely to be good. All you need do is keep an eye out to make sure you're getting enough of the following key players in your diet:

- Vitamin A: Found in orange and yellow fruits and vegetables such as carrots and pumpkins, and fish oil
- Beta carotene: Orange, yellow and green fruits
- Vitamin C: Citrus fruits, green leafy vegetables (such as broccoli), cauliflower, strawberries, raspberries and blackberries, potatoes and sweet potatoes
- Vitamin E: Nuts, seeds, vegetable oils and oily fish
- Selenium: Brazil nuts, tuna, cabbage
- Zinc: Sunflower seeds, fish, almonds.

The best way to make sure is to eat five portions of vegetables a day, and three of fruit. But don't panic – it's not as hard as it sounds!

A vegetable *portion* is 1 to 2 cups of raw vegetables, or 1 cup cooked.

A fruit portion is 1 medium apple or banana. (Fruits are nutritional powerhouses as well, but we limit them more than vegetables on the Protection Plan because some fruits (such as sugar-rich bananas or raisins) can raise insulin levels if you don't eat them with a protein, like a handful of nuts. All-fruit meals can upset your blood sugar levels and should be avoided.

Don't forget that fresh-pressed juices, smoothies, soups and frozen vegetables all count towards your portions, and you can boost the amount of nutrients you get if you eat them raw whenever possible. Next best is steaming or stir-frying rather than boiling (if you do boil your vegetables, keep the nutrient-rich water or stock to use in soups and casseroles).

PHYTOESTROGENS

Phtyoestrogens – plant oestrogens – are chemicals found in plant sources that mimic the action of the body's own oestrogens but on a much weaker scale. There are three main classes of phytoestrogens:

1. Isoflavones – the richest source of all, found in legumes such as lentils, chickpeas and soya beans
2. Lignans – found in nearly all cereals and vegetables, with the best source being linseeds
3. Coumestans – found mainly in alfalfa and mung bean sprouts.

You'll also find phytoestrogens in many everyday foods (see page 98).

How do phytoestrogens work?

Phytoestrogens are not the same as the oestrogens your body produces, but they do have a similar chemical structure. 'Within each cell in the body you have an oestrogen receptor site, which is a little space like a space for a key in a lock,' says UK nutritionist Maryon Stewart, founder of the Natural Health Advisory Service. 'During your menstruating years your oestrogen levels are high enough so that the sites are satisfied by circulating oestrogen. The problem is that when oestrogen levels fall at the time of the menopause, the sites are not satisfied and they remain empty, so they will take whatever oestrogen they can get. For instance, if there's nothing else going these receptor sites will take xenoestrogens, which are carcinogenic environmental oestrogens that come from pesticides, plastics and environmental waste. Phytoestrogens prevent this happening because they take the place of natural oestrogens instead.' And because they give out a weak oestrogenic signal, they act like a natural HRT, replacing the lost oestrogen from your body with a weaker version that encourages hormonal balance and therefore reduces your symptoms.

Studies show that phtyoestrogens can increase oestrogen levels when too low, and reduce them when they are too high.[3] This could explain why soya, a rich source of phytoestrogens, can reduce hot flushes for women going through the menopause (when it's thought that there's an oestrogen deficiency) and protect against breast cancer (often due to an excess of oestrogen).

How many phytoestrogens do you need?

Opinions vary as to how many phytoestrogens you need daily in order to get the most benefit. 'The recommended amount is about 45 mg of isoflavones a day,' says Dr Marilyn Glenville, 'And how long it takes before the effects are felt vary from woman to woman. It depends on how severe your symptoms are and how healthy you are to start with. It would normally be about 4 to 8 weeks.' As well as helping to balance hormones and beat PCOS symptoms, phytoestrogens have a protective effect on cardiovascular health. Studies show that they can lower the level of bad (LDL) cholesterol.[4] It's also thought they may contain compounds believed to inhibit breast and endometrial cancer.[5] Further studies have shown that soya can improve bone density and reduce cholesterol levels, helping to protect you from osteoporosis and heart disease into the bargain.[6]

Because phytoestrogens have a balancing effect on your hormones they are an important part of the Protection Plan diet guidelines – particularly if you've irregular periods.

Action plan for including phytoestrogens in your diet

- Eat plenty of vegetables, in particular green leafy or cruciferous vegetables such as broccoli, cabbage and Brussels sprouts, which have been shown to have not just hormone-balancing but anti-cancer properties.[7] Phytoestrogens are found in almost all vegetables.
- Eat plenty of legumes. Phytoestrogens are most beneficial in the form of isoflavones, found in soya, lentils and chick peas. Beans are easy to use and are great added to soups, salads and casseroles. Hummus is a dip made from chick peas and is available ready-made from most supermarkets or easy to make on your own (see recipe, page 266).
- Although soya products have had some bad press (there has been concern about aluminium levels in soya which have been linked to Alzheimer's), eaten in moderation – say three or four times a week – they can be good for women with PCOS. Eat soya in its traditional form choosing products such as miso, tofu or organic soya milks, and avoid gimmicky snack bars unless they are made from whole soy beans.

Other sources of phytoestrogen include almost all fruit, especially apples, plums, cherries, cranberries and citrus fruits, grains such as rice, oats, barley, rye and wheat, seeds including linseeds, sesame, pumpkin, poppy, caraway and sunflower, and some herbs including cinnamon, sage, red clover, hops, fennel and parsley.

PROTEIN

We've stressed the importance of protein in a PCOS diet, and of eating it alongside any sugary or high-GI snacks to slow down the conversion of sugar by your body. Giving yourself a protein check from time to time is a good thing to do, not only as protein plays its part in maintaining blood sugar balance but also because protein gives your body an even supply of the amino acids it needs to build and repair cells and manufacture hormones and brain chemicals. Protein also helps to mobilize stored fat for use as fuel, thus keeping insulin levels lower. Since your body can't store proteins, as it does carbohydrates and fats, you need a constant supply. That's why you need to eat some high-quality protein with every meal.

But make sure you don't go too far the other way. With the current craze for low- and no-carbing, many people are eating too much protein. Excess protein isn't wise for long-term health if you've got PCOS (although if you need to lose weight fast and you're doing it under medical supervision, a low-carb diet can be a helpful short-term measure). If you fill up on proteins you've less room for nutrient-rich foods that can help balance your blood sugar levels and boost your energy levels. Following a high-protein regime could also lead to raised cholesterol levels, which in turn can trigger diabetes. Diabetes specialist Dr Jim Mann of the University of Otago, New Zealand, claims that high-protein diets create a resistance to insulin. Instead we recommend eating some good-quality protein with each meal, as it's crucial for the metabolism of fat and hormonal balance,[8] while making sure you're also eating the right kind of nutritious carbs as part of a varied and balanced diet (for more information on the right kind of carbs, see Chapter 10).

- For blood sugar control, a sensible balance is two portions of carbohydrate to every one portion of protein. One portion of protein = half a cup of baked beans, 2 eggs, 3 ounces of cheese or three-quarters of a cup of cottage cheese.

- Try to include a range of protein in your diet, with a serving at every meal in the form of low-fat cottage cheese, ricotta cheese, quark cheese, low-fat milk, yogurt, lean meat, poultry, seafood, fish and eggs.
- Other excellent sources of protein are soybeans, split peas, kidney beans, peas, wheat germ, lima beans, black eyed peas, lentils, black beans, spirulina and grains such as quinoa, wholegrain cereals, soy products, tofu products and quorn, as well as nuts and seeds (also good sources of EFAs).
- Try to eat at least two or three eggs a week; five if you're a vegetarian. Eggs are high in cholesterol but because your body doesn't absorb it this cholesterol will not fur up your arteries. They are also high in protein and in lecithin, a superb biological 'detergent' capable of breaking down fats so they can be used by your body – very useful for women with PCOS. Lecithin also prevents the accumulation of too many toxic substances in the blood and encourages the transportation of nutrients through cell walls. Eggs should be soft boiled or poached, since a hard yolk binds the lecithin, rendering it useless as a fat detergent.

FIBRE

You probably think of fibre in terms of the effect it has on your bowels – and actually, a lot of the women we've spoken to who have PCOS and have felt sluggish, have reported constipation as a common problem. But fibre also plays an important part in balancing your hormones, so it can help to tackle PCOS at its source. The fibre contained in grains and vegetables reduces oestrogen levels and seems to prevent excess oestrogens from being reabsorbed into the blood. Studies show that women who eat a high-fibre diet are able to excrete three times as many old oestrogens (hormones the body doesn't need any more) as women who eat meat as well.[9] Meat-eaters' bodies are less efficient at excreting old oestrogens.

Tips for vegetarians and vegans

If you are a vegetarian or vegan, your best plan of action is to seek advice from a doctor or nutritionist (see the Useful Contacts chapter for some suggestions). Meanwhile here are some quick tips for ensuring you get enough protein:

- If you're the only vegetarian in your house, make sure you substitute pulses, beans, wholegrain cereals, dairy products, tofu products or quorn instead of just omitting the meat part of meals you prepare for the rest of the family.
- Nuts, seeds, grains, pulses, soya and vegetables are good sources of protein. Try to eat 30g of nuts and seeds a day.
- Eat plenty of fruits and vegetables.
- Choose cereals fortified with vitamins, particularly B_{12}. Yeast extracts are also good sources of B_{12}. A good multivitamin and -mineral is essential.
- Try to eat a large portion of green leafy vegetables each day and at least half a pint of semi-skimmed milk to ensure your calcium intake. If you're lactose intolerant you can get your calcium from soy milks and yogurts.
- Eat dried fruits, pulses, green vegetables, and whole grains for fibre and iron. Dark chocolate is a good source of iron, too.
- Try to eat at least four eggs a week.
- Choose margarine or butter spreads fortified with vitamin D and E.

Studies have shown that switching to a vegetarian diet can reduce levels of harmful LDL cholesterol. However, similar effects can be seen just by reducing the red meat in your diet to once or twice a week, switching to fish and poultry and avoiding saturated (animal) fats.

There are many long-term problems associated with excess oestrogen, including obesity, heart disease and breast cancer, but also immediate problems including fatigue, weight gain, mood swings and low libido, so plenty of fibre in your diet is important for right now as well as for the long term.

Fibre slows the conversion of carbohydrates into blood sugar, thus helping to maintain blood sugar balance. Dr James Anderson at the

University of Kentucky showed that diabetes control is greatly enhanced by eating a high-fibre diet.[10] In his study, people with Type II diabetes ate a diet composed of wholegrain cereal, vegetables and legumes; their fibre intake was 50g a day. After only a few weeks on this programme, many subjects experienced better glucose control and were able to cut back on their diabetes medication.

If you don't eat enough fibre, PCOS symptoms like weight gain, raised cholesterol, blood sugar problems, insulin resistance and excess oestrogen are likely to get worse. So think about what you're eating and just check it's giving you the best amount of fibre.

You should aim to eat around 30 to 50g of fibre a day. As a rough guide, an apple has about 2g and an orange about 3g.

If you eat your five portions of vegetables and three portions of fruit a day, you're well on the way towards your fibre intake. You can get the rest from complex carbohydrates such as wholegrain cereals, nuts and seeds.

It's best to avoid bran, which acts too fast and prevents you absorbing nutrients.

Legumes such as beans and peas are a good source of fibre and good for blood sugar control. Research suggests that they may also be important for lowering cholesterol and preventing cancer.[11] One study reported in the medical journal the *Lancet* showed that people with Type II diabetes who ate a cup and a half of legumes a day for six weeks had a 15 per cent reduction in fasting blood glucose levels and a 15 per cent reduction in cholesterol.

Drink plenty of water to help fibre pass through your system. And if you aren't used to a high-fibre diet you need to introduce it slowly to give your bowels time to adapt. Don't be surprised if you pass more bulk the more fibre you eat.

HERBS AND SPICES

Herbs and spices have been used to flavour food and to treat various diseases and ailments for thousands of years. Spices are derived from the roots, bark, buds and fruit of plants, while herbs are usually taken from the leaves of various plants. Both herbs and spices are excellent antioxidants, which as you know work to neutralize attacks made by free radicals against the body. Spices also contain phytonutrients, which may prevent the mutation of healthy cells into cancerous cells. Most herbs, especially rosemary, sage, oregano, thyme and onions, have significant amounts of flavonoids which can act as antioxidants to protect LDL cholesterol from being oxidized, and can inhibit the formation of blood clots and provide anti-inflammatory and anti-tumour activity. Studies have shown that a higher intake of flavonoids is linked to lower incidence of heart disease and stroke.[12]

So herbs don't just add flavour and colour to meals (for suggestions on how to use them more in order to add flavour and help you lower your salt intake, see pages 85–87), they appear to play a role in the prevention and management of heart disease, cancer and diabetes – and as such are of particular benefit to women with PCOS.

It would be impossible to list all the beneficial herbs and spices, but here are a few that are of particular benefit to women with PCOS:

Cinnamon

Cinnamon is used to control the level of blood sugar for people with diabetes. It's also used to relieve the symptoms of urinary tract and yeast infections. Studies in rats have shown that cinnamon lowers blood glucose and cholesterol levels.[13] A study published in *Diabetes Care* in December 2003 has shown that small amounts of cinnamon in humans can lower blood glucose, cholesterol and triglycerides.[14]

Fennel

Fennel is a herb used widely to treat infant colic and wind. It's also a strong digestive aid, liver-detoxifier and diuretic with anti-cancer properties.

Other herbs that may protect against cancer include garlic, onions, chives, leeks, mint, basil, oregano, sage, thyme, rosemary, parsley, linseed, ginger, turmeric, dill, celery, coriander, fennel, cumin, anise and caraway.

Fenugreek

Fenugreek is used by many women who suffer from symptoms of the menopause – hot flashes, night sweats, etc. It's also used to reduce cholesterol and relieve constipation. Fenugreek is high in saponins and soluble fibre, which help decrease the absorption of cholesterol from food and can help lower blood glucose levels in people with diabetes. Fenugreek appears to lower blood sugar levels by interfering with the digestion and absorption of sugars and by improving the utilization of sugar once it's absorbed. Two studies published in the *European Journal of Clinical Nutrition* reported that fenugreek improves glucose intolerance in people with Type II diabetes.[15] It can therefore help protect against insulin resistance, Syndrome X and diabetes.

A dose of 25 to 50 mg of fenugreek seed powder twice daily with meals appears to be effective. *Caution:* Fenugreek shouldn't be used if you're pregnant.

Other herbs that are thought to help improve glucose control and insulin activity include cinnamon, garlic, onions, bay leaves, cloves, cumin and turmeric.

Garlic

Garlic is one of the best-known and most widely used herbal medicines. It's a strong weapon against infection and a natural antibiotic, and has been found to reduce cholesterol and high blood pressure.

Garlic (half to one clove per day) is thought to lower triglycerides (blood fats) without affecting HDL (good) cholesterol levels, and may be useful for people with mild hypertension.[16]

Garlic also has a sulphur-containing compound called allicin which inhibits the growth of some bacteria, moulds, yeasts (including Candida) and viruses, and has anti-clotting activity by preventing blood platelets from sticking together.

Finally, garlic has been shown to protect against the development of stomach and colon cancer.[17]

Ginger

Ginger has many medicinal uses. It's a very effective treatment for motion sickness and general nausea and menstrual cramps. Ginger contains a number of natural phytochemicals that inhibit the formation of blood clots and help prevent cancer.

Nutmeg

This common household spice is a natural stimulant to the cardiovascular system. It's also used to relieve the joint inflammation associated with gout. Nutmeg should be used carefully, since large doses can be toxic. It's not to be used by pregnant women as a herbal remedy.

Parsley

This attractive and widely used herb is one of the most nutritious garnishes, containing good amounts of vitamin C and iron. Fresh parsley also makes a great breath freshener. Try it after eating garlic.

Rosemary

Rosemary can aid digestion and improve circulation to the brain. It can also help prevent liver toxicity and has anti-cancer properties. It's good for circulatory problems, menstrual cramps and high blood pressure.

Thyme

Thyme can help lower cholesterol levels and is high in vitamin B, which is important for women with PCOS. Other herbs that are thought to lower cholesterol include celery seed, garlic and fenugreek.

Turmeric

Turmeric has been used to boost insulin production and prevent heart disease. It's also thought to strengthen digestion, decongest the liver and improve flexibility by softening tight muscles and joints.

VITAMINS AND MINERALS

Each vitamin and mineral has a different but crucial function in your body. These nutrients are responsible for the millions of chemical reactions that take place to make your body work the way it's supposed to. A diet lacking in essential vitamins and minerals will affect hormonal balance and health, and if you've got PCOS it's important that there isn't any deficiency.

The best way to bring minerals and vitamins into your body is via the food you eat, but because optimal nutrition is so crucial for women with PCOS it makes sense to take a good multivitamin and -mineral every day. 'Good diet is the foundation of good health. However, it takes a while to kick in, and a good multivitamin and -mineral is a great back-up for women with PCOS. All women with PCOS should definitely take one daily,' says Dr Ann Walker, Senior Lecturer in Human Nutrition at the University of Reading.

All vitamins and minerals are essential to hormone balance, good health and well-being, but if you've PCOS certain vitamins and minerals are of particular importance. The following play a key role in easing PCOS symptoms and reducing the long-term health risk of heart disease, diabetes and cancer.

Vitamin B
The B vitamins are very important in helping to correct the symptoms of PCOS. This is because B vitamins are essential for healthy liver function and proper digestion and absorption. If you've got PCOS it's important that your liver functions well. The liver is your body's waste-disposal system, not only for toxins but for hormones as well. If your liver isn't working well you get an accumulation of toxins and old hormones left over from each menstrual cycle which can make your PCOS symptoms worse and increase your long-term health risks.

Your liver deactivates old hormones and renders them harmless. It needs B vitamins to carry out this process. Studies have also shown that giving women vitamin B_6 increases their fertility and helps regulate their menstrual cycle.[18] Research also suggests that several of the other B vitamins figure strongly in blood sugar control.

- Vitamin B-rich foods: lentils, brown rice, whole grains, beans, low-fat dairy products, eggs, nuts, seeds, bananas (B_6), lean meat, fish, fruits and vegetables

Vitamin C

Research has shown that the antioxidant vitamin C helps with the clearance of toxins from the body, improves blood sugar control, lowers cholesterol, boosts immunity and generally promotes a feeling of health and well-being.[19] It can also speed up a slow metabolism and help improve circulation to the scalp.

Vitamin C is an important nutrient for all women and especially for those with PCOS symptoms of insulin resistance, obesity, acne, thinning hair and irregular periods.

- Vitamin C-rich foods: most fruits and vegetables, citrus fruits, potatoes and green vegetables

Vitamin E

Vitamin E is a powerful antioxidant and plays a protective role in the body. Studies have shown that adding the antioxidants vitamin C and E to an animal's diet can balance hormones.[20] As well as boosting immunity, balancing blood sugar, improving skin and hair condition, research has shown that this important vitamin may also play a role in the prevention of heart disease,[21] which is important news for women with PCOS who are insulin resistant. Similarly there's compelling evidence that vitamin E supplements can lower the risk of breast cancer.[22]

- Vitamin E-rich foods: nuts, wholegrain cereals and vegetable oils such as sunflower and wheat germ oil

Chromium

Chromium is an essential mineral which can help lower blood glucose levels. Insufficient chromium intake can make you vulnerable to insulin resistance and diabetes. Several well-documented studies have shown that supplementing with chromium may improve blood sugar control in insulin-resistant individuals.[23] In addition to its role in regulating blood sugar, chromium can help you maintain healthy levels of HDL (good cholesterol) Chromium is also the most widely researched mineral in the treatment of obesity.

- Chromium-rich foods: wholegrains, yeast, rye bread, chicken, cornmeal, bananas, carrots, oranges, green beans, cabbage, mushrooms and strawberries

Iron

An iron deficiency can make symptoms of PCOS worse, in particular irregular and/or heavy periods, hair loss, infertility, fainting and dizziness and fatigue. Apart from eating iron-rich foods, cooking foods in iron cookware or stainless steel and avoiding aluminium pans, and drinking tea with food (tannin in tea can block the uptake of iron) can increase your iron intake.

- Iron-rich foods: fish, poultry, leafy green vegetables and dried fruit

Magnesium

Magnesium strengthens bones, teeth and muscles. It's also essential for energy production as it's used by your body at the very first stage of the process that converts glucose to energy. Studies have shown that there's a strong link between magnesium deficiency and insulin resistance, so it's important if you've got PCOS.[24] For instance, scientists at Harvard Medical School conducted a trial and came to the conclusion that magnesium-rich foods can prevent the development of diabetes.

- Magnesium-rich foods: low-fat dairy products, nuts, seeds, soya beans, whole grains, leafy green vegetables, lean meat, bitter chocolate

Manganese

Manganese is an essential trace element needed for blood sugar balance. People with diabetes can often be deficient in manganese and therefore it's important for women with insulin resistance.[25]

- Manganese-rich foods: whole grains, nuts, beans, fruits and green leafy vegetables

Zinc

Zinc plays an important role in the synthesis, storage and secretion of insulin and is important for women with PCOS and insulin resistance.[26] Zinc also works as an antioxidant by protecting the body's cells from free-radical damage. If zinc levels are low your immune system will not function properly; there could also be problems with your menstrual cycle as zinc is necessary for a healthy reproductive cycle.

Finally, zinc is excellent for problem skin. It helps reduce the inflammation response within the body and aids healing.

- Zinc-rich foods: wholegrains, beans, pulses (beans) nuts, low-fat dairy foods and fish

PCOS-friendly foods

Now you've read about how to make your diet PCOS-friendly, you might be feeling bewildered about precisely which foods you should be eating – or avoiding – day to day. Here's a selection of just some of the kinds of food you can include on your shopping list – you'll see there's plenty to choose from.

- Fruit: Apples, bananas, plums, cherries, peaches, strawberries, raspberries, oranges, grapes, dried fruit, tangerines, currants, grapefruit, pears, dates, figs, watermelon, blueberries
- Vegetables: Cabbage, broccoli, green beans, mushrooms, celery, cucumber, carrots, potatoes, sweet potatoes, lettuce, parsley, spinach, watercress, asparagus, beetroot, Brussels sprouts, cauliflower, peppers, tomatoes, turnips, edible seaweed (kelp)
- Legumes: Soya beans, butter beans, mung beans, chick peas, haricot beans, green and brown lentils, garden peas, low-sugar baked beans, kidney beans, split peas, black eyes peas, beansprouts, alfalfa beans
- Seeds: Sunflower, sesame, hemp, pumpkin, linseed, flax
- Nuts: Almonds, cashew nuts, Brazil nuts, pecan nuts, walnuts
- Grains: Wholewheat flour, quinoa flour, brown rice flour, rye flour, barley flour, buckwheat, millet, rice, oats, oatbran, wholemeal bread, granary bread, wholegrain pasta, brown rice
- Dairy: Low-fat skimmed milk, eggs, low-fat yogurt, low-fat cottage cheese, ricotta cheese, unsalted butter – non-dairy alternatives such as goat's, sheep and soya milks and cheeses
- Meat and fish: Oily fish (salmon, sardines, mackerel, tuna) chicken, turkey, lean red meat – non-meat alternatives such as soya, tofu, tempeh
- Herbs and spices: Garlic, turmeric, ginger, cinnamon, onion, fennel, fenugreek, rosemary, thyme, tarragon, sage, nutmeg, parsley
- Vegetable oils: olive oil, flaxseed oil, wheat germ oil, hempseed oil, soy oil, coconut oil, peanut oil
- Sweet treats: Home-made ice cream from skimmed milk with no added sugar, dark chocolate, low-fat spreads, low-fat muffins, wholemeal scones, rice cakes, oat cakes, sesame crackers
- Freshly-squeezed fruit juices and smoothies

**SAMPLE
MENUS**

Right now the seven-day meal plan outlined below may seem very different from what you're used to eating, but please don't let this worry you or put you off. The plan includes the sorts of meals you're aiming to be eating regularly once you've worked through all the stages of the Protection Plan. (See also the PCOS-friendly recipes beginning on page 265.)

Drinks aren't mentioned in the menu plans, but it's important to get plenty of water, herbal teas and fresh fruit and vegetable juices. (Take your multivitamin and -mineral first thing in the morning with some organic fresh-pressed apple or other fruit juice.) All bread should be wholegrain; pre-packaged foods should contain as few additives as possible and, if you can, make sure your fruit and vegetables are organic.

Note: In addition to breakfast, lunch, dinner and the two snacks in between, you may want to add a small snack such as fruit and a handful of nuts and seeds or a glass of low-fat milk and an oatcake just before bedtime.

Day one
- *Breakfast:* Two slices of wholemeal toast with peanut butter, glass of low-fat milk
- *Mid-morning:* Handful of mixed sunflower seeds and almonds
- *Lunch:* Wholemeal pitta bread with lean chicken and salad or hummus and salad, bowl of berries with low-fat yogurt
- *Mid-afternoon:* Three dried apricots and three cashews
- *Dinner:* Steamed fish or tofu with steamed brown basmati rice and stir-fried vegetables

Day two
- *Breakfast:* Two boiled eggs with wholegrain toast, piece of fresh fruit
- *Mid-morning:* Carob bar (you can get these from health food shops)

- *Lunch:* Big bowl of salad with tomatoes, green leaves, herbs such as basil, olives, nuts, onions, feta or other grated cheese; fruit tartlet with walnuts
- *Mid-afternoon:* Handful of mixed dried fruit and nuts
- *Dinner:* Mixed vegetable home-blended soup with toasted sesame and pumpkin seeds, with a lean chicken or seafood or veggie sausage sandwich

Day three
- *Breakfast:* Oat porridge with linseed, raw honey and rice milk
- *Mid-morning:* Banana and a handful of walnuts
- *Lunch:* Mixed vegetable casserole, an apple
- *Mid-afternoon:* Three dried apricots and three walnuts
- *Dinner:* Tuna or cheese salad with two wholemeal rolls, low-fat ice cream with crushed almonds

Day four
- *Breakfast:* Fresh fruit salad sprinkled with hemp seeds, two slices of wholemeal toast
- *Mid-morning:* Dried fruit and sesame seed crackers
- *Lunch:* Lean meat or fish, medium jacket potato, large helping of vegetables or salad, apple
- *Mid-afternoon:* Vegetable sticks with low-fat cottage cheese
- *Dinner:* Scotch broth, hot fruit compote with low-fat yogurt

Day five
- *Breakfast:* Two scrambled eggs, 2 slices rye bread
- *Mid-morning:* Apple, handful of nuts
- *Lunch:* Mixed bean and vegetables casserole with wholegrain rice, bowl of raspberries sprinkled with cashews and low-fat yogurt topping
- *Mid-afternoon:* Two rice cakes with low-fat cottage cheese and cucumber

- *Dinner:* Baked wild salmon with potatoes, broccoli and carrots, fresh fruit and almonds

Day six
- *Breakfast:* Fresh fruit salad topped with low-fat yogurt and sesame seeds
- *Mid-morning:* Banana and a handful of nuts
- *Lunch:* Large bowl of vegetable soup with lean turkey or low-fat cheese salad sandwich
- *Mid-afternoon:* Cup of strawberries and low-fat ice cream
- *Dinner:* Wholemeal pasta, broccoli, red onion and tomato salad with garlic and lemon juice, small bar of dark chocolate.

Day seven
- *Breakfast:* Grilled sardines or low sugar baked beans on two slices of wholemeal toast
- *Mid-morning:* Pear and a handful of nuts
- *Lunch:* Tuna or cheese salad with jacket potato, bowl of raspberries with cashews and low-fat yogurt topping
- *Mid-afternoon:* Banana and sesame seed crackers
- *Dinner:* Mixed vegetable casserole, strawberry and dark chocolate mousse

If there are any meals in this plan that you just can't imagine yourself eating on a regular basis, don't worry. A long-term diet needs to be practical and sustainable, and you should feel free to use your imagination to find recipes and food combinations that you enjoy and can prepare easily. Use our suggested recipes (beginning on page 265) and try swapping tips and ideas with other women with PCOS over email groups or on the Internet.

SIMPLE RULES

We'll finish this section with some basic rules to both recap and help your body make the most of the nutritious food you're feeding it.

Make changes gradually

Making changes to your diet takes a lot of effort and perseverance. If you're used to eating a lot of sugar, salt, fat and chemical flavourings, your taste buds will be loath to make drastic changes. That's why we recommend that you give yourself time to adjust to the new flavours and appearance of food in its more natural form. With determination your tastes will change and, as your symptoms start to ease, you'll find that it gets easier and easier. You can of course start eating new foods immediately, but this could trigger headaches, lethargy and diarrhoea as your body detoxes. It's far better to avoid this shock to your system with gradual changes and to train your palate and digestion slowly. It takes about three to six months for most people to adjust to any new eating programme.

Watch your portion size

Eating more than you need will lead to weight gain, which isn't good for women with PCOS. Proper attention to serving size will ensure that you get your nutrients but not the extra calories. Portion sizes have got bigger over the years, and waistlines have followed suit.

If you aren't sure how much you need, the daily servings guidelines from the US Department of Agriculture can help:

- 2–3 servings of meat, fish, eggs, beans, nuts a day
  1 serving = one egg, half a cup of beans, or meat or fish about the size of a deck of cards
- 2–3 servings of milk, yogurt, cheese or non-dairy produce such as soya
  1 serving = 2 oz of cheese or 1 cup of milk or yogurt
- 4–6 servings of wholegrains

1 serving = 1 slice of bread, half a cup of rice or pasta, bowl of cereal
- 4 servings of fruit
  1 serving = 1 piece of fruit
- 5 servings of vegetables
  1 serving = half a cup of raw or cooked vegetables
- fats and oils in moderation

Start checking your portion size, and if need be make a few small reductions. You don't need to cut down on your favourite foods, just eat less of them.

Protein and carbohydrates at every meal

Carbohydrates give you energy. Protein has a stabilizing effect on the sugar released from carbohydrates into the blood, producing steady, long term energy instead of short bursts followed by a let-down that can trigger excess insulin and PCOS symptoms.

Simple carbohydrates (apart from fruit) are all refined foods where all the goodness is stripped away. They cause a rapid rise in blood sugar which can lead to an excess of insulin. The difference between the effects of the simple and complex carbohydrates on the body is enormous. Unlike simple carbohydrates, complex, preferably low-GI carbohydrates (wholegrains, vegetables) are far better for women with PCOS because they can lower cholesterol and help balance blood sugar and hormones.

Don't eat a big meal after 8 p.m.

The typical way many of us find ourselves eating is a small or non-existent breakfast followed by a light lunch and then a big evening meal. Sometimes people don't eat at all until their evening meal, which can be as late as 8.30 p.m. Stacking your calories like this isn't a very good idea if you've got PCOS, because if you hardly eat during the day your metabolic rate slows and your body does its best to hold on to every last calorie. Then when you eat in the evening your body is set to store as much fat as possible. After eating you then often go to bed so your body has little time to use any of the calories you've just consumed. To sum up, eating late confuses your metabolic rate and encourages weight gain, which isn't helpful if you've got PCOS.

Get snacking

The best way to eat if you've got PCOS is little and often. Start the day with breakfast, have a mid-morning snack, followed by lunch, a mid-afternoon snack and dinner. By spreading your calories throughout the day, not only do you give your body and mind the energy they need to function optimally but you also keep your blood sugar stable. If there's a long gap between meals, your blood glucose drops too low, adrenaline is released to get your liver to produce more glucose to rectify the imbalance, and you end up with too much glucose in the blood. Your body is then on a roller-coaster ride of fluctuating blood sugar levels which can only make your PCOS symptoms worse.

Cut down on the Ss and increase the Fs

When you're choosing what to eat, cut down on sugar, salt and saturated fat and increase your intake of fluids, oily fish and oils.

Plenty of fruits and vegetables

Vegetables and fruits are essential for women with PCOS. As well as helping to balance hormones, the fibre in fresh vegetables and fruit helps to regulate insulin levels. Try to eat fresh, raw fruit and veg, as these are likely to have the highest nutrient content and highest enzyme activity. Enzymes are to your body what batteries are to a car. Overcooking often destroys life-enhancing enzymes, so when you do cook vegetables, steaming them lightly or stir-frying them are the healthy alternatives.

Make sure you've got lots of colour on your plate

A useful trick is to think of the colours of the rainbow when you choose your fruit and veg. A good selection of colours means that you're getting a good selection of nutrients. So aim for multicoloured meals – check orange, green, yellow, red and purple are all present by choosing foods such as cabbage, peppers, carrots and blackberries. The deeper the colour, the more nutrients are present.

Nuts and seeds every day

Seeds, such as sunflower, sesame, hemp and pumpkin are packed with nutrients that can help boost your health and well-being. They can be eaten as they are, sprinkled over salads and cereals or used in baking. Flax, pumpkin and sesame are particularly useful as they contain phytoestrogens. Nuts, too, should be included in your daily diet. All nuts are nutritious, but almonds, cashew nuts, Brazil nuts and pecans offer the greatest amount. Walnuts are good as they are high in oestrogen. Eat a wide assortment as snacks, with cereals and in baking.

A variety of grains

Aim to eat a wide variety of grains. Oats are highly recommended because they can help stabilize blood sugar levels. Avoid fortified and refined flours as they have little nutritional value. Healthy flours to include in your diet include wholewheat or wholemeal, quinoa, oat, maize, rye, barley, potato and brown rice flour – all of which are high in nutrients. Buckwheat, millet and rice aren't grains but they make good alternatives. Wheatgerm is high in vitamin B, and as such it's highly recommended for women with PCOS. When choosing bread, the word 'brown' in the description means nothing – check to see if wheat and rye grains have been added.

Remember the 80/20 rule

In general, the more nutritious and natural (nothing added or taken away) your food is, the better – but don't set yourself up for failure. You can't eat healthily 100 per cent of the time. The occasional treat – bar of chocolate, bag of chips, pastry – doesn't mean you've failed. It's the extremes that are potentially harmful to your health. No food is completely off-limits in the PCOS Protection Plan diet. It's important to eat healthily most of the time, but also to enjoy your food and allow yourself the *occasional* indulgence.

> **66***After four years of missed periods, facial hair and being overweight I decided it was time to see my doctor. He examined me and said I may have polycystic ovaries. I was like "poly what?" Anyway, I was told I had insulin resistance and sent to a diabetes centre to learn about diet. Common sense really, like making sure I get enough fibre, get all my nutrients and don't eat foods that might trigger blood-sugar swings. What was new for me was the "little and often" advice. I've always been a three-square-meals-a-day woman.*
>
> *I made the changes suggested and also started walking to work instead of taking the bus. The first month was really hard and I nearly gave up. I thought I must be getting full-blown diabetes as I was constantly tired and needed to go to the restroom all the time, but my doctor told me this was my digestive system adjusting and it would clear up soon. He was right. It did. When I went back to the doctor in about three months I had lost some weight and was feeling better. And in six months not only did the weight loss continue but my periods returned. Today I'm doing great. I still get the occasional blip if I don't take care of myself, but I know how to get back on track. I sometimes feel angry that I have to be so healthy, but then I remind myself of how good it feels to be healthy and proud of the way I look.***99**

Laura, 38

REFERENCES

1. Chan, J. *et al.*, 'Water, other fluids, and fatal coronary heart disease', *Am J Epidemiol* 2002 Jan; 155 (9): 827–33
2. Fenkcv, I. *et al.*, 'Decreased total antioxidant status and increased oxidative stress in women with polycystic ovary syndrome may contribute to the risk of cardio-vascular disease', *Fertil Steril* 2003 Jul; 80 (1): 123–7
3. Barnes, S. *et al.*, 'Soy isoflavones – phytoestrogens and what else?', *J Nutr* 2004 May; 134 (5): 1225S–1228S

4. Stark, A. *et al.*, 'Phytoestrogens: a review of recent findings', *J Pediatr Endocrinol Metab* 2002 May; 15 (5): 561–72

5. McCann, S. E. *et al.*, 'Dietary lignan intakes and risk of pre- and postmenopausal breast cancer', *Int J Cancer* 2004 Sep 1; 111 (3): 440–3; Horn Ross, P. L. *et al.*, 'Phytoestrogen intake and endometrial cancer risk', *J Natl Cancer Inst* 2003 Aug 6; 95 (15): 1158–64

6. Hanna , K. *et al.*, 'Phytoestrogen intake, excretion and markers of bone health in Australian women', *Asia Pac J Clin Nutr* 2004; 13 (Suppl): S74; Altavilla, D. *et al.*, 'Cardiovascular effects of the phytoestrogen genistein', *Curr Med Chem Cardiovasc Hematol Agents* 2004 Apr; 2 (2): 179–86

7. Keck, A. S. *et al.*, 'Cruciferous vegetables: cancer protective mechanisms of glucosinolate hydrolysis products and selenium', *Integr Cancer Ther* 2004 Mar; 3 (1): 5–12

8. Andersson, U. *et al.*, 'AMP-activated protein kinase plays a role in the control of food intake', *J Biol Chem* 2004 Mar 26; 279 (13): 12005–8

9. Gerber, M. *et al.*, 'Fibre and breast cancer', *Eur J Cancer Prev* 1998 May; 7 Suppl 2: S63–7

10. Anderson J. W., Bryant, C. A., 'Dietary fiber: diabetes and obesity', *Am J Gastroenterol* 1986; 81: 898–906

11. Shi, J. *et al.*, 'Saponins from edible legumes: chemistry, processing, and health benefits', *J Med Food* 2004 Spring; 7 (1): 67–78

12. Nowicka, G. *et al.*, 'Flavonoids: antioxidative compounds and their role in prevention of ischemic heart disease', *Pol Merkuriusz Lek* 2003 Nov; 15 (89): 441–4

13. Khan, A. *et al.*, 'Cinnamon improves glucose and lipids of people with type 2 diabetes', *Diabetes Care* 2003 Dec; 26 (12): 3215–18

14. Ibid.

15. Madar, Z. *et al.*, 'Glucose-lowering effect of fenugreek in non-insulin dependent diabetics', *Eur J Clin Nutr* 1988 Jan; 42 (1): 51–4

16. Wilburn, A. J. *et al.*, 'The natural treatment of hypertension', *J Clin Hypertens* (Greenwich) 2004 May; 6 (5): 242–8

17. 'Eat your garlic!', *Integr Cancer Ther* 2002 Dec; 1 (4): 422–3

18. Kidd, G. S. *et al.*, 'The effects of pyridoxine on pituitary hormone secretion in amenorrhea–galactorrhea syndrome', *J Clin Endocrinol Metab* 1982; 54 (4): 872–5

19. Krajcovicova, K. M. *et al.*, 'Free radical disease prevention and nutrition', *Bratisl Lek Listy* 2003; 104 (2): 64–8

20. Tarin, J. *et al.*, 'Effects of maternal ageing and dietary antioxidant supplementation on ovulation, fertilisation and embryo development in vitro in the mouse', *Reprod Nutr Dev* 1998 Sep-Oct; 38 (5): 499–508

21. Kartal Ozer, N. *et al.*, 'Molecular mechanisms of cholesterol or homocysteine effect in the development of atherosclerosis: Role of vitamin E.', *Biofactors* 2003; 19 (1–2): 63–70

22. Kline, K. *et al.*, 'Vitamin E and breast cancer', *J Nutr* 2004 Dec; 134 (12 Suppl): 3458S–3462S

23. Kleefsha, N. *et al.*, 'Chromium and insulin resistance', *Ned Tijdschr Geneeskd* 2004 Jan 31; 148 (5): 217–20

24. Lopez, R. R. *et al.*, 'Magnesium intake and risk of type 2 diabetes in men and women', *Diabetes Care* 2004 Jan; 27 (1): 134–40

25. 'Concentrations of seven trace elements in different hematological matrices in patients with type 2 diabetes as compared to healthy controls', *Biol Trace Elem Res* 2001 Mar; 79 (3): 205–19

26. Salguerio, M. J. *et al.*, 'Zinc and diabetes mellitus: is there a need of zinc supplementation in diabetes mellitus patients?', *Biol Trace Elem Res* 2001 Sep; 81 (3): 215–28

12 Lifestyle Changes for Body and Soul: Exercise, Detox, Stress-busting

EXERCISE

66 *Not all women with PCOS are going to want to jog and weight-train for hours every day, and we don't need to. What we do need to do is get more active. We all just need to move, whether it's gardening, yoga or walking. Exercise can change our lives. It has changed mine. I've never felt healthier.* 99

Sally, 31

66 *I've tried every diet there is — you name it and I've done it. Some worked better than others but soon the weight starts creeping slowly back. Even eating like a rabbit does not make me lose weight and I've come to the conclusion that for women with PCOS, like me, the only way to lose weight and keep it off is to eat healthily and to exercise. It's easier to exercise than to diet, and exercising with friends is not only inspiring, it's fun. I suggest that you start slowly and with something you enjoy, rather than something you hate — like 10 minutes' walking and then build up to an hour. Lose a bit of weight first before you start anything more complicated, or you might get injured or find you can't do it and give up. If you want to go to the gym, go at off-peak times until you feel more confident — there's nothing more demotivating than watching skinny girls strut their stuff in skin tight gear.* 99

Gillian, 32

The benefits of exercise for women with PCOS just can't be exaggerated.

Recent research confirms that regular, moderate exercise has a direct effect on controlling your hormones.[1] Exercise in combination with a healthy diet is one of the most natural, effective and healthy ways to combat PCOS,[2] helping with just about every symptom.

We know that extremes of exercise alter the menstrual cycle dramatically – women athletes, for example, sometimes don't have periods at all – so it's thought that moderate, routine exercise suppresses the production or over-production of hormones. Women who engage in regular exercise have fewer PCOS symptoms than those who don't because exercise can help achieve proper insulin levels – and when insulin levels are controlled, this helps control testosterone and oestrogen levels.

Exercise helps to keep your bowels working efficiently to eliminate waste products and hormones your body doesn't need. It boosts immunity and helps to improve thyroid function, which has a direct effect on metabolism. It helps you look and feel better. When you exercise, brain chemicals called endorphins are released which boost mood and help you feel happier and calmer. Studies have shown that exercise can also have a positive effect on women suffering from stress, anxiety, insomnia, fatigue and depression.[3]

There's another very important reason why exercise is such a crucial part of the Protection Plan: it can help protect you from the long-term health risks associated with PCOS.[4] Not only does activity add vitality to your years by improving your health and outlook on life, it adds years to your life by reducing your chances of developing chronic diseases like diabetes and heart disease. Researchers from the Cooper Institute in Dallas, Texas have found that women who are fit are at a lower risk of developing diabetes relative to women of lower fitness. The researchers suggest that doctors prescribe physical activity to their female patients to help prevent the development of the disease.

Proven benefits for long-term health risks
Insulin resistance and diabetes
Recent research confirms that regular, moderate exercise can lower blood sugar levels and promote insulin efficiency.[5] Studies of women with diabetes have shown improvements with blood sugar control after only one week of aerobic exercise – and just one bout of exercise boosts insulin sensitivity for 16 hours or longer. Exercise lowers your blood sugar levels by burning it as fuel, and the fitter you are, the lower your body fat and the better your insulin and glucose control.

Heart disease
Exercise increases circulation and also seems to lower LDL (bad) cholesterol and increase HDL (good) cholesterol levels.

High blood pressure
Studies show that exercise can help to reduce high blood pressure.[6]

Syndrome X
Exercise is an integral part in the treatment and prevention of metabolic syndrome.[7]

Obesity
Regular exercise in combination with a healthy diet is one of the most effective ways to combat obesity. Not only does exercise burn calories, it can also help speed up your metabolism and balance your hormones so you're less likely to gain weight. Studies show that if you're fit you burn more calories even while you're resting, because it takes more calories to maintain muscle tissue than fat tissue. So the more you exercise, the more your muscles build up and the speedier your metabolism becomes – making it easier for you to lose weight if you've got weight to lose.

There's another reason why exercise is such a great weight-loss tool: it can distract you from food and help curb your appetite by modifying in a positive way the activity of the hormones that regulate appetite.

Women who exercise regularly find that they're less likely to get food cravings or feel constantly hungry.

Breast and endometrial cancer

High levels of oestrogen in the blood can instigate the growth of hormone-sparked cancers such as breast and endometrial cancer, so it makes sense that if hormone levels are more balanced through healthy diet and exercise, then the risk is reduced. Research has shown how beneficial exercise can be in the prevention and treatment of breast cancer.[8] A study reported in the US *Journal of the National Cancer Institute* has shown that women who exercise for around four hours a week have a 58 per cent lower risk of breast cancer, and those who exercise for between one and three hours a week had a 30 per cent lower risk. In the UK's Nurse's Health Study, which has followed a group of more than 20,000 students since 1976, women who exercised for 7 hours a week or more were nearly 20 per cent less likely to develop breast cancer than their more sedentary sisters.

Osteoporosis

Exercise is also crucial for your bones because it can help to keep up a good level of bone density. If you make few demands on your bones, you'll be risking osteoporosis. Even moderate exercise has been shown to increase bone density in post-menopausal women.[9] Placing demands on your bones (through weight-bearing exercise, for example) encourages them to maintain their density.

Your exercise prescription

Your exercise routine will depend on your general health, your age and any health conditions you may have. If you haven't exercised for a while, are over 40, have high blood pressure and/or insulin resistance and are overweight, your first step is to check with your doctor for safety guidelines.

Once you know it's safe to exercise, exercise safely! Use your common sense and listen to your body. Obviously when you first get going there will be some discomfort or even soreness after a session, but there shouldn't be any pain, fainting, dizziness, shortness of breath or nausea. So don't overdo it. If something doesn't feel right, STOP immediately and consult your doctor.

Be sure to wear loose, comfortable clothing when exercising, and make sure your shoes offer the correct support. Drink plenty of water before, during and after your workout even if you don't feel thirsty, and have light snacks on hand to help if you get a sudden dip in energy.

Finally, pay attention to your breathing when you're exercising. Try to prevent it becoming quick and shallow. You should breathe in deeply through your nose and out through your mouth.

To improve your health and quality of life you don't need to join a gym or run the marathon, you need just 30 minutes of activity per day. And you don't have to get all 30 minutes at once – it can be spread throughout the day and can include activities such as:

- climbing stairs
- a brisk walk
- house-cleaning
- walking while on your mobile.

All activity counts. You just need to get 30 minutes a day most days of the week.

If you don't think you're getting your 30 minutes, find ways to get there: park further away from work so you've got to walk, take the stairs instead of the lift, carry your shopping home, wash your car by hand, mow the lawn. In the long run these simple changes can help you prevent health complications and feel better about yourself.

Picking up the pace

Once you're in a routine of getting 30 minutes' activity a day, it's time to pick up the pace in the Protection Plan – with aerobic exercise.

Aerobic exercise is any exercise that involves rhythmic motion of your arms and legs — walking, jogging, swimming and so on — that temporarily increases your breathing rate. Ideally you should aim for aerobic exercise for 20 to 60 minutes three to five times a week, but if it's all new to you start with 10 minutes three times a week and build from there. If you're overweight or have high blood pressure, again make sure you check with your doctor first.

Why include aerobic exercise? Because it improves your body's ability to use insulin. It can also strengthen your heart and lungs and help you manage your weight. A good exercise routine that you can repeat daily, every other day or three times a week, would look something like this:

- 5 to 10 minutes of gentle warm-up exercises to increase your heart rate gently.
- Moderately-paced aerobic exercise that works the large muscles and elevates your heart rate for 20 to 30 minutes. The aim is to get your heart rate up to 60 to 75 per cent of its maximum capacity (220 minus your age). You should feel slightly out of breath but not so much that you can't carry on a conversation.
- A cool-down period that includes stretching exercises to improve your flexibility and range of motion.

Fast walking is an ideal form of aerobic exercise, but you may prefer jogging, cycling, an exercise class or swimming. Whatever you decide, make sure you enjoy it. Studies show that exercise drop-outs often punish themselves with exercise routines they don't enjoy. So if you hate jogging or swimming, don't do it. If dancing, rambling, horse-riding or boxing are things you enjoy, make them part of your exercise routine. You may also want to ask your partner or a friend to exercise with you. When you exercise with other people you're more likely to continue because you can motivate each other and because it's tougher to break a commitment to exercise if you're doing it with someone else.

Finally, if you do skip a workout, don't let it derail your exercise prescription. If you're working out five times a week for 30 minutes each time, giving yourself a day or two off now and again isn't going to undo the good you've done.

Strengthen your routine

In addition to your aerobic exercise you'll also need to include some strength-bearing activities two or three times a week. The more muscle you've got, the more calories you burn and the better your blood sugar and insulin balance even when you're not exercising. Good muscle tone will make you look fitter as well as protecting your joints from stress.

Walking and cycling are good weight-bearing exercises, but strength training is even better. The aim isn't to turn you into a weight-lifter – you only need to do two sets of repetitions, like press-ups which work your upper body and squats which work your lower body. You can go to your gym and ask for a individualized programme, but if you can't face the gym or it isn't an option, some 3- to 8-lb dumb bells (or two tins of soup) can give you the benefits.

To get the most out of weight training you need to make sure the exercises are performed correctly, so it might be worth investing in an instructional video or book.

Strengthen your motivation

You may find it hard to motivate yourself to exercise on a daily or regular basis, but consider this: if you've got PCOS, exercise is as important as diet in reducing the long-term health complications such as diabetes, high blood pressure, obesity and heart disease. An exercise programme – even one as simple as 15 to 30 minutes' walking a day – can significantly reduce all these risks.

66 *I'm on the Pill – I have abnormal periods if I'm not. I get acne, hair on my face and my stomach, and severe water retention. I'm 20 pounds*

overweight. I also have hypertension. It wasn't until I started to check out some PCOS websites last year that I found out I wasn't alone and I have a real reason for being overweight. I have found a new doctor who is giving me advice about diet and exercise in combination with metformin, and things are looking up. I'm also talking to friends and family more about PCOS and everyone is on my side. I'm talking a multivitamin and -mineral and my acne and facial hair have definitely improved. I've also lost 9 pounds. Finding out there were other women like me, enlisting the support of family and friends, making grown-up choices about food and making my life more active have made a huge difference. I'm still not completely sane yet, but I'm feeling hopeful for the first time in years. I'm unsure if this is all because I finally know what's wrong with me — it isn't all my fault, I have PCOS and this may partly explain why I sometimes feel so lousy — or because I have started to pay attention to the food I eat and the exercise I do, but I feel much better. With everything we "cysters" have to watch out for — heart problems, diabetes, infertility — it's good to think that I'm not helpless and there are things within my control. 99

Kristin, 40

WEIGHT MANAGEMENT

66 *Like clockwork, every time I get even just a little overweight my symptoms come back to remind me that I've got PCOS.* 99

Lily, 36

66 *Why can't I lose weight? People don't believe me when I say I eat like a bird, but I really do. I'm not bingeing in private. Is PCOS making me fat?* 99

Janice, 18

Being overweight can trigger PCOS symptoms and insulin resistance, and significantly increase your already increased risk of long-term health complications. 'Weight reduction remains the best way for women with PCOS to reduce the risk of diabetes and the complications associated with it in the long term,' says PCOS expert Professor Stephen Franks, Professor of Reproductive Endocrinology at Imperial College, London.

Weight-management is a really positive step for women with PCOS, but as we've seen, insulin resistance and the slower metabolism that go with PCOS can make weight loss incredibly hard. So what can you do if you if you've tried diet after diet and nothing works?

Escaping the PCOS weight trap

❝ *My doctor told me that if I lost weight my PCOS symptoms would get much better, but I really don't eat that much. Sometimes I indulge in the odd take-away, but on the whole I don't think I eat more than anyone else. I really think that being overweight is natural for me. It's just the way I am.* ❞

Sue, 21

❝ *Losing weight is very hard for me. No sooner have I put something in my mouth than it appears on my hips and bottom. I've tried every diet but never lose more than a few pounds.* ❞

Louise, 33

❝ *I started to diet when my best friend said she wanted to lose weight. We decided it would be fun to motivate each other. We exercised together and compared our diets and they were very similar, but although my friend whittled herself down to a size 10, I actually put on a few pounds. I think for many women with PCOS the weight gain is the biggest challenge. There doesn't seem to be an answer. I'm tired of everyone looking at me and thinking that I must be secretly bingeing. I really am not. How do I win the battle?* ❞

Sarah, 43

The first essential step is to eat a PCOS-friendly diet like the one we've outlined earlier. This will help stabilize your blood sugars. Then, add in some regular exercise to help lower blood sugar levels, balance hormones, speed up your metabolism and reduce cravings. The next step is to start adding things on top of your basic diet-and-exercise programme to help you lose weight: getting motivated, cutting your portion size, fighting food cravings and taking food supplements.

Motivation

One of the biggest problems with weight loss is motivation. It's all very well saying you should lose weight to protect your health, but it's easy to get bored or put things off. For most of us, life needs to get really uncomfortable before we break out of our familiar routines, so if you're reading this book and still can't get motivated, here are some tips to help you.

Keep a food diary

Keeping a food diary can help because it puts the focus on you. It forces you to think about whether your diet is helping your symptoms or making them worse. A food diary gives you a feeling of control, but the most important thing about writing down what you eat is the awareness it brings and the way it encourages you to notice what you're doing. You can't change habits you aren't aware of.

Make a contract with yourself

You could also draw up a contract with yourself to change your eating and exercise routines in ways that can help you become slimmer and fitter. A contract with yourself may sound odd, but research shows that writing down your goals and aspirations makes them more real and helps you stay focused on achieving them.[10]

Visualization

Knowing that you need to lose weight or wishing that you could lose weight isn't the same as making the decision to lose weight.

Motivational techniques, such as visualization, can help you get in touch with what you really want. Try this one.

- Close your eyes and imagine yourself 20 years older. In all those 20 years you haven't made any healthy changes to your lifestyle. Now imagine what you'd look like and how you'd feel. Would you feel (and look) old and tired? How much weight have you put on? What would your health be like? Would you have aches and pains? Would you get out of breath walking up a flight of stairs? Would you still be able to put shoes and stockings on with ease?

Such techniques can be a bit of a shock to the system, but they help you bring focus and commitment to your weight-loss plan.

If the threat of diabetes, heart disease and poor health in the future doesn't seem real enough now, why not give some thought to what else might motivate you? It's OK if improved health and preventing the onset of chronic disease aren't your primary motivations for losing weight. There are many other benefits. What about appearance? Feeling better? Looking toned and sexy? Finding muscles you didn't know existed? Keeping up with your kids in the park? Dropping a dress size?

One of the best ways to motivate yourself to make changes in your lifestyle is to think about *all* the benefits you'll gain when you lose weight. No matter how silly or vain they may feel, write them down. This will help you see up front what you stand to gain if you start taking steps to manage your weight. Let this list motivate you, re-energize you and keep you going.

Portion control

One of the most effective ways to cut back on the calories without skimping on the nutrients is portion control. (For a refresher on portion size, see page 114.) You don't need to cut out your favourite dishes, you just need to eat less of them. If you think that smaller portions won't satisfy your hunger, there are things you can do to give you that full feeling:

- Take time over your meals. Put your knife and fork down after each mouthful and chew your food slowly.
- If you still feel hungry, wait 10 or 15 minutes. It takes quite a while for your brain to recognize that your stomach is full.
- Never shop or cook when you're hungry. Keep a supply of healthy, low-fat, low-sugar snacks to hand, such as apples and nuts, dried fruit and low-fat yogurts, and remember the 'little and often' rule so you never get really hungry.
- Give your body food every few hours to boost your metabolic rate and keep blood sugar levels stable. Around six meals a day is best for losing weight and for keeping hunger at bay. If there's a long gap between meals, blood sugar levels fall too low, leaving you tired, craving sugar and lacking in energy and concentration.
- Stop eating several hours before you go to bed. A light snack is OK – say a cracker and a glass of low-fat milk if you feel peckish – but don't have a heavy meal. This is because your body needs to rest, not digest, while you sleep. The earlier in the day you eat, the more likely you are to burn off calories, even if you aren't active.
- Make nutrient-rich foods such as whole grains, fruits and vegetables the staples of your diet. They're filling but low in calories.

Beat food cravings

66 *I've been diagnosed with PCOS and I know I need to watch my weight, but sweets are my downfall. If there are chocolates or biscuits around, I simply can't resist. Sometimes I get such strong cravings I have to drive to the shops in the middle of the night. I'm not insulin resistant (although if I carry on like this I surely will be), but I am very overweight and get horrible outbursts of acne.* 99

Mary, 22

Many women with PCOS find that they have strong sugar and carbohydrate cravings, and this plays havoc with their weight-loss plans. Sugary carbohydrates such as cakes, chocolate, sweets and pastries are the foods we often crave because they send blood sugar levels rocketing, giving us an instant energy boost that is, unfortunately, short lived as it leads to an overproduction of insulin followed by a dip in blood sugar, leaving us tired and sleepy and craving sugar all over again.

If you suffer from food cravings, all the healthy eating tips listed above will help keep them at bay – but you can really help yourself by using the glycaemic index when making your carbohydrate food choices. If you want to eat a food with a high GI, make sure you balance it with some protein and fat to slow down the release of sugar. Dr Barry Sears, creator of the Zone diet which has proved useful for women with PCOS, urges women with PCOS to ensure every meal has a good balance of carbohydrate, protein and fat to moderate insulin levels and keep you feeling fuller for longer.

If your food cravings lead to food binges and comfort eating, you aren't alone. As many as 75 per cent of women who have weight to lose struggle with binge-eating. This problem is so common that it has been diagnosed by medical professionals and been given a name – binge-eating disorder.

Bear in mind that there's a difference between binge-eating and the odd bout of overeating now and again. If binges happen several times a week and you feel out of control, you probably have binge-eating disorder. If you even suspect you've got this problem, you need to seek help. Why? Because all the positive lifestyle changes and weight-management that our Protection Plan recommends can be counteracted by binge-eating. You need to address this disorder separately from your efforts to lose weight; the best people to seek advice and help from are your doctor, a counsellor or a registered dietician. They will help you get your bingeing under control by focusing on the underlying issues that trigger it. Once you're better able to manage the bingeing, you can look forward to real success with weight loss.

Food supplements

All nutrients are important, but when it comes to weight loss certain nutrients are more important than others. If you're deficient in any of these, it could hinder your weight-loss plans. We've listed the major supplements that may be able to help you lose weight, but it's important to point out that they can only be effective alongside a healthy diet according to the Protection Plan guidelines.

B vitamins

B vitamins are important for weight loss because they are involved in energy production and help to control fat metabolism and help you digest your food better.[11] If digestion is good you're more likely to use your food efficiently instead of storing it as fat. It's best to get your B vitamins from your diet (foods such as wholegrains, nuts, fish, vegetables and low-fat dairy produce are rich in B vitamins), but if you think you may be deficient the best way to make sure you're getting enough vitamin B is a good B complex supplement.

Chromium

Chromium is needed for the metabolism of sugar; without it, insulin is less effective in controlling blood sugar levels. This means it's harder to burn off food as fuel and that more is stored as fat. It may also help control levels of fat and cholesterol in the blood.[12] Good food sources of chromium include whole grains, bananas, carrots, cabbage, mushrooms and strawberries. If you want to supplement, most people take 50 to 200mcg a day of organic chelated chromium picolinate rather than standard chromium supplements, which are less easy to absorb. Dr Ann Walker recommends 600 mcg of chromium GTF for women with PCOS who are insulin resistant.

Manganese

This mineral helps with the absorption of fats and also works to stabilize blood sugar levels. It also functions in many enzymes, including those involved in burning energy. Foods rich in manganese include green leafy vegetables, pecans, pulses and whole grains.

Magnesium

Magnesium aids in the production of insulin and helps to regulate blood sugar levels.[13] Foods rich in magnesium include green leafy vegetables, nuts and seeds and soya beans. If you want to supplement with magnesium, the recommended daily intake is in the region of 300 mg.

Co-enzyme Q10

Co-enzyme Q10 is needed for energy production. Studies have also shown that it can help with weight loss.[14] Good food sources include sardines, soya oil, whole grains and mackerel. If you want to supplement, ideally it should be taken under the guidance of a nutritional therapist; the usual daily dose is two 60 g capsules twice a day.

Zinc

This is important because it can help control appetite. A deficiency can make you lose your sense of taste and smell. Make sure that your multivitamin and -mineral contains zinc, and include more zinc-rich foods in your diet such as green leafy vegetables, nuts, seeds, whole grains and eggs. If you don't think you're getting enough zinc, you may want to take a daily 15–g supplement – but no more than this as high levels can make you vulnerable to infection.

Other nutritional supplements often recommended to help lose weight include:

- potassium and calcium – important in the production of energy
- EFAs (essential fatty acids) – for appetite control
- psyllium husks – for fibre to promote a fuller feeling
- kelp – contains minerals that can help with weight loss
- lecithin capsules – can help break down fats
- spirulina – can help stabilize blood sugar
- vitamin C – to speed up a slow metabolism
- boron – speeds up calorie-burning (raisins and onions are good sources)

- the amino acids L-ornithine, L-arginine and L-lysine — research has shown that taking these in combination can improve weight-loss efforts.

Apart from your daily multivitamin and -mineral, if you want to take any supplements you should consult your doctor or a nutritional therapist first. You also need to remember that supplements won't help you a great deal unless you are also eating a healthy diet and exercising regularly.

If you want to take any herbal or fat-fighting supplements to help you lose weight, such as Siberian ginseng, fennel or fenugreek, you also need to make sure you consult your doctor and a trained dietician or nutritionist first. Certain herbal supplements can be toxic in large doses. And unless your doctor feels that your weight carries a serious risk to your health, steer clear of slimming drugs of any kind. What you need is permanent weight loss; the drawback of slimming drugs is that they are like crash diets: they don't work in the long term.

Set a realistic goal

Setting yourself a weight-loss goal depends a lot on your age and circumstances. You may have to settle for 5 or 10 per cent below your current weight — even this would be enough to prevent diabetes and heart disease. If your goal is to lose a great deal of weight — say more than 50 pounds — consider this a long-term goal, something to be accomplished over the next three years. Break it down into manageable stages — aiming to lose 20 pounds a year.

Whatever your goal, weight loss of 1 or 2 pounds a week is a realistic and healthy expectation and sets you on the path to finding your natural weight.

When setting your weight-loss goal, do take your body shape into account. Your weight might be right for you, but where you carry it makes a difference. 'Apples' and 'pears' are definitely not equal when it comes to the risk of developing diabetes and other diseases. If you're an 'apple' (see page 47), the risk is higher.

BMI

How much do you have to lose to prevent diabetes and heart disease? How do you know if you're at a healthy weight?

The best tool we have at present for deciding if you're at a healthy weight is the BMI – body mass index. Essentially, the BMI is a formula that relates to body fat, and it's better at predicting the risk of disease than body weight alone.

If you want to know your BMI, multiply your weight in pounds by 700 and then divide this by your height in inches squared.

BMI = weight x 700 divided by height x height.

For example, if you weigh 200 pounds and are 5 ft 7, your BMI would be 31 (200 x 700 divided by 67 x 67, or 140,000 divided by 4,489). If the result of your number is between 19 and 25, you're at a healthy weight and your goal should be to maintain it. A number of 27 or higher is an indication that you're overweight and at higher risk for many diseases.

The BMI can also be used to help you determine your weight-loss goal. If your BMI is over 25, calculate the weight you would need to be to have a BMI of 25 (25 x your height x your height divided by 700). Then subtract your answer from your current weight to find your weight-loss goal.

Do bear in mind that the BMI doesn't take body shape, gender or build into consideration, so can sometimes be only a rough guide. For more information, visit www.bbc.co.uk/health and click on the BMI calculator.

In the months and years ahead you might want to continue measuring your hips and waist – and other parts of your body, too – every few weeks. It's a good way to keep track of your progress and a good alternative to the scales. As you start to lose weight you'll find inches decreasing in almost every area – although in some areas such as your chest and arms, you may find an increase in muscle. By using the tape measure you'll be pleasantly surprised at the toned, fit body that's emerging, and it will decrease your dependence on the scales as a measure of success.

Natural diet boosters

If you've got weight to lose, the best thing to do is eat healthily and exercise regularly according to the Protection Plan guidelines. This will help you get your blood sugar levels balanced so your body is less likely to store sugar as fat. Eating regularly – say three main meals and three snacks a day – is also crucial. 'Don't skip breakfast,' says Marilyn Glenville, nutritional therapist and author of *Natural Alternatives to Dieting*.

- 'Eating breakfast fires up your metabolism so that you end up burning more calories. Make sure you eat regularly as this gives your body the message that there's a plentiful supply of food, so that there's no need for it to store food.'
- A good night's sleep is important, too, as lack of sleep disrupts your hormones, triggering changes in metabolism so that you're not processing food as well as you should. It's thought that lack of sleep is linked with higher levels of cortisol, which can throw your metabolism out of balance. Other studies have shown that lack of sleep can have a negative effect on carbohydrate metabolism and endocrine function, lowering glucose tolerance and making it more difficult to convert carbohydrates into energy.[15] This makes it more likely that fats and sugars are stored as unwanted extra pounds. Further studies have established a link between lack of sleep and increased appetite.[16] It is thought that lack of sleep boosts levels of leptin – a hormone that triggers appetite.
- Drinking four cups of green tea each day is also said to help you lose weight. Studies at the American Society for Clinical Nutrition found that one of its compounds, catechol, increases metabolism and reduces the amount of fat your body absorbs by as much as 30 per cent. Green tea is rich in natural antioxidants which fight the damaging effects of free radicals. These include vitamin B_5, which plays a key role in the body's metabolism, and vitamins B_1 and B_2, essential for releasing energy from food.

- Drinking a glass of water before you eat can also aid weight loss because you'll feel fuller. Water helps to flush out toxins and waste, and helps break down fat. Water can also have a direct impact on energy: we may reach for a sugar fix when what we need to do is rehydrate the body.

- Research has shown that eating chillies or hot peppers can boost your metabolism and reduce your appetite. A study in Melbourne found that volunteers who added red pepper to their diet ate fewer calories. 'They whiz up your metabolic rate by a hefty 25 per cent,' says Dr Caroline Shreeve, author of *Fat-burning Foods*. 'Chilli, cayenne and pepper and mustard should all hit the spot.'

- An increasing number of studies show that cinnamon contains substances which can help the body convert sugar into energy so it's less likely to be stored as fat. Studies by the US Department of Agriculture's Human Nutrition Research Centre in Beltsville, Maryland, found that MHCP (methylhydroxy chalcone polymer, the most active compound in cinnamon) makes cells more responsive to insulin and reduces blood sugar levels by a fifth.

- Scientists in San Diego, California claim you can lose almost a pound a month by adding grapefruit to your usual meals. They monitored 100 overweight volunteers, asking a third to eat half a grapefruit before a meal, a third to drink a glass of grapefruit juice and the other third to avoid grapefruit. After 12 weeks, the grapefruit group had lost an average of 3.6 pounds, the juice group 3.3 pounds and the last group nothing. 'Including grapefruit in your diet can be really helpful,' says Marilyn Glenville. 'Grapefruit reduces insulin levels, which in turn leads to a reduction in body-fat stores.' But Marilyn warns: 'If you're on medication, check with your doctor first as grapefruit can slow the drugs being metabolized by your system.'

- Having a bowl of soup may also help you lose weight. US researchers at Johns Hopkins University in Baltimore found that people who chose soup as a starter consumed 25 per cent less fat in the main meal to follow.

Slow but steady is the key

If you look back at page 138 you'll see that all the natural weight-loss boosters listed above can be found in the Protection Plan diet and healthy living guidelines. Making diet and lifestyle changes is the most successful way to lose weight, but it takes time – typically a good three to six months – before you'll start to see the benefits.

There isn't a quick fix to weight loss. You need to edge slowly and steadily toward your goal. If weight loss isn't immediate, it can be tempting to crash-diet, but faddy diets never work in the long term as they slow your metabolism. The only way to lose weight safely and keep it off for the long term is that healthier eating and exercising regularly become a way of life.

Finally, there's no point in deciding you're going to be ultra-strict so you end up living like a hermit and having no fun. Food and exercise are such an important part of life, you've got to enjoy it. You need a way of eating and living that allows you to be healthy without feeling deprived.

❝I was diagnosed with PCOS very early – I couldn't have been more than 16. My doctor put me on the Pill to sort out my irregular periods. Within a year the weight started to pile on. Not just a few pounds, but stone after stone after stone. I also had facial hair – sideburns and a small beard – which were very noticeable. I felt horrible. My doctor changed the Pill I was on, but this made things even worse. I tried to stay positive and keep my "chins" up, but soon I was shaving my face every day and out of a job because I was taking too much time off due to exhaustion.

'Things changed for the better when my old doctor left and a new one referred me to a dietician with experience of designing diet-and-exercise programmes for women with PCOS. I didn't hold out much hope, as like many women with PCOS I'd tried diets and slimming clubs before without success. My dietician told me that the reason I was finding it hard to manage my weight was that PCOS was slowing down my metabolism. It *was a real eye-opener — for the first time in 10 years, here was someone who wasn't blaming me for being overweight. She personalized a PCOS diet for me based on my slow metabolism and blood sugar problems. To my amazement, I lost 16 pounds in six weeks.*

'I've been working with her for nearly a year now and am a stone away from my target weight. I feel terrific. I'm never hungry or craving food because I eat every few hours to help my metabolic rate keep up. My acne has also cleared. I'm also taking saw palmetto and have seen a definite improvement with my facial hair. I feel a different woman to the woman I was all those years ago.

I'm living proof that PCOS doesn't have to mean a lifetime of weight problems. You don't have to feel helpless. There are things you can do to help yourself. At my worst I was over 20 stone, which was massive for my 5 ft 3 frame. I'm now just under 14 stone. If I can do it, anyone can.

Martha, 28

DETOXING

Although the word 'detox' probably makes you think of whacky weight-loss plans that everyone rushes to try after Christmas, what *we* mean by detox is trying to avoid unnecessary chemicals and pollutants that clog up your system and make it harder for your body to work efficiently. It means you helping your body to feel healthier, and not wasting time getting rid of toxins when it could be repairing itself and running on top form. What's more, many of today's man-made chemicals have been proven to have hormone-disrupting effects — as if we haven't got enough disrupted hormones to deal with already! So, detoxing is actually a really sensible approach to your lifestyle if you have PCOS — your body has enough to cope with without adding a load of waste matter into the mix!

What are toxins?

Every day we're surrounded by potentially hormone-disturbing toxins from the chemicals in everything from plastics to solvents and adhesives, additives, colourings, pesticides and preservatives in foods, chemicals that get into our skin and bodies via our make-up, nail varnish, shampoo, moisturizers and deodorants – not forgetting chemicals like chlorine and the medications that pass into the water we drink. A recent report found traces of Prozac and at least seven other drugs in the UK water supply; there are petrochemicals in pesticides, plastics and household cleaners, and the air we breathe contains pollutants such as car exhaust and cigarette smoke.[17]

Our bodies don't need these chemicals and toxins, and have to work very hard to metabolize them and get rid of them. In the process of metabolizing toxins, our bodies lose vital nutrients that we need to feel healthy, maintain a healthy body weight, prevent disease and beat the symptoms of PCOS. For example, the body needs vitamin C to get rid of the toxins in cigarette smoke.

Natural and unnatural toxins

A toxin is any substance that's detrimental to cell functioning and the optimal health of your body. This includes substances like carbon dioxide in the air or the free radicals our bodies produce as a by-product of producing energy, or the waste we produce through digestion or after fighting off an infection, and also excess hormones our bodies don't need. Your skin, liver, kidneys and adrenal glands work very hard to process these substances and keep you healthy.

On top of this natural toxic load, our bodies have to deal with more and more toxins in the environment. It's estimated that since the 1950s, more than 3,500 new man-made chemicals have found their way into the foods we regularly eat. This puts a huge burden on your liver, kidneys, adrenals and skin. These are the major culprits:

- chemicals and additives in food
- addictive substances that have little or no nutritional value such as tea, coffee, alcohol
- over-the-counter medications
- heavy metals such as lead, cadmium and aluminium in industrial processes, petrol, cooking utensils, domestic water pipes, dental fillings, cigarette smoke, old paint work and antacid medication
- pollutants from carpets, cleaning materials, insecticides, gas boilers, insulation materials, paints, washing machines and car exhausts
- electromagnetic fields (EMF) from TVs, mobiles, microwaves, fridges and electric clocks
- EDCs or xenoestrogens – see below.

Xenoestrogens

Xenoestrogens, or endocrine-disturbing chemicals (EDCs), are chemicals found in pesticides or plastics that are widely recognized as highly toxic even in the smallest doses. Most importantly for women with PCOS, they are classified as hormone-disruptors because they have a molecular structure similar to that of oestrogen.

As soon as they enter your body, either through your mouth, nose or skin, EDCs interfere with your hormones and prevent them from doing their job correctly. They may occupy or alter oestrogen-receptor sites in tissue cells, or interfere with the manufacture of oestrogen by the ovaries or adrenal glands. Some mimic oestrogen in the body while others block oestrogen's effects, tricking your body into a condition known as oestrogen dominance or oestrogen excess.

We don't know enough about EDCs yet, but we do know that for some reason they love fat. They are stored in body fat, and overweight people tend to have higher concentrations.[18] For women with PCOS, who are often struggling with weight issues, any xenoestrogens we take in will more than likely find a place to set up home.

If you're exposed to high levels of oestrogen anyway because irregular ovulation leaves you without the balancing effect of progesterone, the presence of xenoestrogens can trigger oestrogen dominance and PCOS symptoms such as bloating, abdominal weight gain, fatigue, irregular periods and a number of health problems, from dry skin to an increased risk of heart disease, infertility and even cancer. If no ovulation occurs there's no progesterone to counteract the effects of oestrogen, and a hormonal imbalance results.

> Oestrogen and progesterone counter each other's effects in a normal menstrual cycle. Oestrogen stimulates uterine lining and breast cell growth, and promotes water retention. It's also associated with an increased risk of breast cancer and insulin resistance. Progesterone stabilizes uterine and breast cell growth and helps the body burn fat as fuel. It has been credited with fighting heart disease, insulin resistance, cancer and osteoporosis.

There's no doubt that women with PCOS are affected by xenoestrogens, which may also be at the root of some of the health complications associated with PCOS.[19] For example, research has shown that women with higher concentrations of certain EDCs in their bodies run a greater risk of developing breast cancer than women with lower levels.[20] A startling discovery was made by Professor Ann Soto in Boston, Massachusetts. She was studying breast cancer cells stored in large incubators and discovered that the cells began to divide and multiply as if oestrogen were present. When she changed the test tubes, the cells stopped dividing. It turned out that nonylphenol, a synthetic oestrogen similar to those widely used in toiletries, skin creams, agricultural chemicals and detergents, had been used in the manufacture of the test tubes and was being leached into the breast cell culture, causing the cells to be stimulated. Think about the implications if the creams you use on your body contain this chemical! (See page 152 for ideas on using chemical-free toiletries.)

Your in-house detoxifying system

Your body has its own in-house detoxifying system to remove toxins.

The major player here is the liver. Your liver is a chemical cleaning workaholic that neutralizes and removes toxins and excess hormones such as oestrogen and sends them to the kidneys for elimination. Alcohol, fatty foods, highly refined foods, smoking, drugs, EDCs and other environmental toxins can overload your liver and, when levels are too high, clog your liver's pathways. When this occurs blood sugar levels start to fluctuate, excess hormones can't be cleared and PCOS symptoms get worse. The strain on your liver will force your other detoxifying organs (your skin, lymph system and kidneys) to work overtime, which can cause rashes, acne, testosterone excess, bloating, yeast infection and poor general health.

Are you suffering from toxic overload?

Signs of toxicity are diverse, and differ from person to person. The following are the most common signs and symptoms of excess toxicity:

- bad breath
- sore or coated tongue
- fatigue
- headaches
- weight gain
- bowel and digestive problems
- allergies
- high cholesterol
- blocked arteries
- skin disorders such as acne or rashes
- gall bladder problems
- a wide variety of mental symptoms – your brain is not capable of disarming toxins and is heavily dependent on your liver to do so. If your liver isn't working properly due to toxic overload it can lead to memory loss, problems concentrating, drowsiness, inability to focus, woolly-brain syndrome and a heightened response to alcohol.

Clearly toxicity is bad news for PCOS sufferers. It can overload your liver, make your symptoms worse and further increase your risk of heart disease, diabetes, obesity and cancer. So what can you do about it?

Protecting yourself from EDCs and toxic overload

Detoxing can help with blood sugar control, and by so doing help protect against hormonal imbalance, diabetes, obesity, heart disease and possibly breast cancer. There are countless detox programmes and diets recommended for cleansing your system, but they aren't usually a good idea as they slow your metabolism and are hard to stick to.

You don't really need to go on fasts, retreats or harsh regimes, or take supplements to protect yourself from toxicity. The best way is to keep your body's own self-purifying system in good order by giving your liver, kidneys and adrenals nutritional support, reducing your exposure to toxins and following our top-20 detox recommendations.

1. Follow the Protection Plan guidelines for a healthy diet

Nutrients can help your liver process, transform or eliminate toxins and excess hormones. A healthy diet can help you prevent, control and repair the damage toxins have caused, while working to restore hormonal balance in your body.

Detox superfoods

Certain foods are thought to strengthen and improve liver function, support the kidneys and adrenals, and so aid detoxification.

For the liver
- apples
- asparagus
- berries
- broccoli
- brown rice
- buckwheat
- cabbage

- carrots
- celery
- fennel
- garlic
- kelp
- leeks
- lemons and lemon juice
- millet

- oat bran
- oily fish
- onions
- parsley
- parsnips
- quinoa
- sesame oil and seeds
- spices such as dill, mint, tarragon and thyme
- spinach
- strawberries
- sunflower seeds
- teas: alfalfa, burdock, chamomile, dandelion, green, lemon, red clover and rose hip
- turmeric
- watercress

For the kidneys
- asparagus
- beetroot
- blackberries
- broccoli
- cabbage
- celery
- cranberries
- eggs
- fennel
- garlic
- grains such as buckwheat, barley and millet
- grapes
- green beans
- kidney beans
- leeks
- lettuce
- melons
- oranges
- oysters
- parsley
- peas

- pulses
- raspberries
- sea vegetables
- sesame seeds
- tarragon
- teas: cinnamon, goldenrod, cloves, buchu, nettle and parsley
- turnips
- walnuts
- watercress

For the adrenals
All foods that strengthen the kidneys will also strengthen the adrenals. In addition, it's important to consume foods high in potassium such as bananas, raisins, peanuts, garlic, chicken and carrots, and to avoid foods high in sodium.

Foods high in vitamin C such as apples, oranges and green vegetables are also recommended, as this vitamin is crucial for the production of adrenal hormones.

To boost your detox make sure your multivitamin and mineral complex includes enough vitamin B complex, vitamin C, vitamin E, selenium and zinc. Other nutritional supplements to support the liver include:

- glutamine
- lecithin
- cysteine
- taurine

– but these should only be taken under the guidance of a nutritional therapist.

2. Get more fibre
Fibre can help prevent the absorption of oestrogen chemicals into your bloodstream.

3. Eat more cruciferous vegetables
These include broccoli, Brussels sprouts, cabbage and cauliflower. Not only can they help prevent disease and poor health, they are high in substances called indole-3-carbinol which help to prevent toxic oestrogen from being absorbed in the body, while at the same time encouraging its elimination.[21]

4. Eat phytoestrogens
Foods such as soya, lentils and chicken can naturally reduce the toxic forms of oestrogen in your body and help prevent the risk of diseases such as hypertension and breast cancer.[22]

5. Reduce your intake of saturated fats and transfats
There are two reasons for this. First of all you'll minimize the fat stores that present a welcome home for xenoestrogens and the toxic burden that brings, and secondly a high intake of saturated fats and transfats is directly linked to obesity and heart disease.[23]

6. Avoid plastics
Avoid as far as possible food and drinks in plastic containers or wrapped in plastic. Don't store any fatty foods (cheese, meat, etc.) in plastic wrap. Because xenoestrogens are lipophilic (fat-loving), they will tend to leach into foods with a high fat content. Remove food from plastic wrapping as soon as possible and don't heat food in plastic.

7. Try to go organic
As much as possible, buy organic fruits and vegetables. There are thousands of types of insecticides, herbicides and fungicides approved for use in the UK and US, and some fruits and vegetables are sprayed as many as 10 times.

8. Drink pure water

The World Health Organization has claimed that 80 per cent of the world's illnesses would be eliminated if we drank pure water. It's estimated that as many as 60,000 different chemicals, metals and toxins now contaminate our water supply. Ideally you should purify drinking water in the home with a water filter jug, readily available from department stores and health food shops. Alternatively, buy bottled water (in glass, not plastic) or drink boiled then cooled tap water (boiling it first gets rid of bacteria and lime scale). If you're still drinking tap water and suspect you've got lead pipes, use only cold water for drinking and cooking.

9. Avoid sugar and salt

The body sees these substances as unwanted toxins that increase your risk of hypertension, heart disease, diabetes and cancer. Processed, ready-cooked, tinned and refined foods are often packed with salt and sugar, and are high in additives (see below). Watch out, too, for alternative names. For instance, sodium is another name for salt, animal fat is saturated fat and sugar has many pseudonyms: sucrose, fructose, dextrose or maple syrup, to name but a few. If you're following the whole food diet approach of the Protection Plan, you'll be well on the way already.

10. Axe the additives

Food additives have been linked to a variety of health problems, including headaches and allergies.[24] For women with PCOS, these additives – colourings, preservatives, flavour enhancers, stabilizers and thickeners – add to your toxic load and make symptoms of PCOS worse by blocking the body's own detox system. Highly refined foods tend to have substances added to enhance flavour and prolong life; these additives are known to be harmful to health and upset hormonal balance.[25] As hormone levels in PCOS are already abnormal, further upset can only make things worse. The additives that cause the most damage are monosodium glutamate (MSG), colourings (look for E numbers on the label), sorbate, sulphates, aspartame, butylated hydroxyanisole and butylated hydroxytoluene. As a rule of thumb, if you can't understand a label, can't see any natural ingredients or the list of chemical ingredients is so long there's barely enough room, leave it on the shelf.

11. Cut down on caffeine

Coffee, tea and chocolate all contain caffeine. Caffeine gives you an energy boost but at the same time over-stimulates the adrenals and, if you consume too much, weakens them. A cycle develops where greater amounts are needed to give you a high and symptoms such as headaches and indigestion occur if you don't get your fix. If you've got PCOS, too much caffeine can deplete your body of essential nutrients, disturb your sleep and trigger problems with blood sugar.[26] Caffeine has also been linked to irregular periods and infertility.[27] You don't need to cut down altogether, as research suggests that a moderate amount of caffeine does not significantly compromise your health (tea, for example, contains substances that can help protect against heart disease) but you do need to make sure that you don't drink to excess. One or two cups of caffeinated drinks a day seems to be OK, but no more than that. Why not try fruit or herbal teas instead? If you've been heavily dependent on caffeine you may experience withdrawal symptoms for a few days when you start to cut back. If headaches occur, increase your water intake and keep eating a healthy balanced diet. This should ease withdrawal symptoms.

12. Limit your alcohol intake

Alcohol contains a lot of sugar, and because alcohol molecules are so small they are absorbed very quickly into your bloodstream, causing rapid fluctuations in blood sugar which can increase your risk of insulin resistance and diabetes. Alcohol also converts quickly to fat, increasing the risk of obesity and heart disease, and can interfere with normal liver function so it's less able to clear out excess hormones.

The health risks associated with alcohol are directly related to the amount you drink. A high risk would be incurred by having more than five drinks daily, a moderate risk by three to four drinks a day, and a low risk by one or two drinks daily. Women with PCOS should limit their intake of alcohol to no more than five drinks a week. Taken in excess, alcohol can increase the toxic load and increase your risk of disease, but a small amount may have some beneficial effects.[28,29] It's thought, for example, that red wine contains bioflavonoids, while beer is rich in vitamin B which can help decrease the risk of heart disease. It's important to point out, however, that research on the health benefits of alcohol is always based on moderate-to-low alcohol intake.

13. Don't overcook it

Avoid overcooking your food, as this can destroy vital nutrients – nutrients you need to fight toxins. Try grilling instead of frying, lightly steam vegetables instead of boiling them, and avoid all aluminium cookware.

14. Stop smoking

Cigarette smoking is the biggest cause of preventable disease. Studies show that passive smoking has its risks, too.[30] Just 30 minutes in the company of smokers can damage your heart by reducing its ability to pump blood, according to research published in the *Journal of the American Medical Association*.[31] Cigarettes contain anti-nutrients and high levels of chemicals, such as cadmium – a heavy toxic metal that can stop the body from using zinc (needed for a healthy menstrual cycle) properly. It's well known that smoking is linked to menstrual irregularities, early menopause, heart disease, cancer and poor health in general. If you're concerned about the long-term health risks of PCOS and you're a smoker, you should consider why you're taking something into your body that increases your risk further.[32] To protect your health in the future, nothing is as effective as stopping smoking completely.

There are many books about quitting smoking; arguably the most successful method is to go cold turkey. Make the decision to smoke your last cigarette. The nicotine will pass out of your system in a matter of days; the challenge then will be to find healthy habits to replace smoking. A healthy diet, regular exercise and pampering yourself a bit can all help you stay strong. Chewing sugar-free gum, drinking water or jumping on the spot are all techniques ex-smokers have used to beat the cravings. If you need something to do with your hands, buy some worry beads, take up knitting – there are plenty of ideas to be found in quit-smoking books and on the Internet.

15. Buy natural cleaning products

These will help you to reduce the number of potentially xenoestro-genic chemicals in your house. Or use the tried-and-tested cleaning methods preferred by your granny: white vinegar and lemon for stain removal, chemical-free liquid soaps and detergents.

16. Use natural toiletries

Scientists are investigating a link between the chemicals in deodorants and anti-perspirants and breast cancer.[33] The answer is to buy chemi-cal-free where you can.

The same goes for make-up, moisturizers, etc. Explore your local health store and reputable on-line health sites to see just how many natural alternatives there are out there: brands such as Jason Natural Cosmetics, Tisserand, The Green People, Desert Essence, and so forth, are all good places to start with.

Tampons, especially super-absorbent brands, may dry the vagina – making the transfer of toxins into the bloodstream easier. Best to try towels instead. If you do need to use tampons, make sure you change them regularly (every four hours or so). Some studies have found that the only type of tampons that did not produce toxins were 100 per cent cotton ones.[34]

17. Go for a walk

At least once a day, try to take a stroll in a park or green place near your home or workplace. Trees give out energizing oxygen. It's also a good idea to have plants in your home and workplace. NASA research has shown that the following plants can extract fumes, chemicals and smoke from the air: peace lilies, dwarf banana plants, spider plants, weeping figs, geraniums and chrysanthemums.

18. Limit electromagnetic exposure

Common-place items in your home – alarm clock, TV, video, DVD – as well as power sockets may increase your exposure to harmful electromagnetic waves. Buy battery-operated clocks and radios, and unplug electrical sockets just before you go to bed. If your work involves sitting in front of a computer screen, make sure you take regular breaks – get up and walk around or get some fresh air – every 30 minutes or so.

19. Destress

If you're under stress – having a bad week at work, not sleeping properly or struggling with making major decisions – signs of toxicity can worsen. This is because stress causes your energy reserves to be channelled away from your body's detoxification mechanisms. The stress-management techniques and sleeping tips in the pages that follow should help here.

20. Exercise regularly

Exercise is a great detoxifier. It boosts circulation, speeds up metabolism, aids digestion, encourages sweating and elimination and clears your mind.

There's no doubt that pollution and toxin levels are rising steeply, but as you've seen there's plenty you can do to help yourself. Healthy eating, regular exercise and avoiding toxins where possible are, more often than not, sufficient to restore health and prevent the risk of health problems in the future.

66*I used to drink gallons of coffee every day. I also smoked and drank wine every lunchtime and evening. Add to that a busy life, no exercise, a poor diet, stressful job and PCOS and you can see why, in addition to weight gain and acne, I suffered from bad breath, fatigue, migraines and dizzy spells. Like many women with PCOS I had no idea that all the toxins I was pumping into my body were making my symptoms worse. It was tough giving up smoking – even tougher giving up coffee and alcohol. It* *was tough cutting back on my work commitments and simplifying my life, but it was all worth it. I have my energy back, my symptoms have vanished and, best of all, I feel 10, even 20 years' younger.* **99**

Laura, 47

SLEEP

How often do you wake up feeling refreshed and ready to take on the day? Sleep is essential to your health and well-being. Most of us, however, burn the candle at both ends, running round trying to do too much in too little time. An estimated 10 to 20 per cent of the population currently experience frequent sleep disruption, according to the Surrey Sleep Research Centre (SSRC). In the words of Dr James Parish from the Sleep Disorder Mayo Centre in Scottsdale, Arizona, 'The Surrey Sleep studies confirm what we have known for a long time: Sleep deprivation is an epidemic.'

If you're well rested both mentally and physically you can cope better with the demands of a busy life. During deep sleep your body stores protein, restores energy levels and is flooded with a surge of growth hormones – important for cell renewal and repair and good health in general. Dreaming while you sleep is a way for your mind to sort through problems in your daily life so that they don't increase your health-damaging stress levels. Even missing a few hours of sleep a night on a regular basis can have a detrimental effect. Life will feel more stressful and you'll be less productive. You may have problems concentrating as well as irritability and, of course, fatigue – not great if you're already feeling sluggish due to PCOS. A recent study has also shown that the number of the body's natural killer (NK) cells, responsible for fighting off bacteria and viruses, is also decreased if you don't get enough sleep (no surprise to those of us who end up with colds when we're run down).[35]

Sleep is particularly important for women with PCOS, because sleep-deprivation not only raises stress hormones, making it harder to cope with the demands of your daily life, research findings show that it disrupts hormonal balance,[36] interferes with blood sugar levels and increases the risk of insulin resistance and diabetes,[37] Syndrome X,[38] high blood pressure, obesity,[39] hypertension[40] and heart disease,[41] and may even be linked to breast cancer.[42] It seems that good quality sleep can also help beat the day-to-day symptoms of PCOS.

How much sleep do you need?

Everyone has different sleep needs, but if one or more of the items on the list below apply to you, you're not getting enough good-quality sleep:

- you yawn a lot
- you fall asleep during the day
- you lack energy
- you feel drained or tired
- you need caffeine and stimulants to get you through the day
- you get dark circles under your eyes
- you find waking up difficult
- you find it hard to concentrate
- you get irritable for no reason.

What is good quality sleep?

Up until recently, eight hours of sleep a night was recommended for optimum health – but it's important to realize that quality, not quantity, is the key. A recent study showed that those who sleep for fewer than six hours or more than seven would experience increased irritability.[43] Seven hours seems to be the most beneficial, but six hours of good quality sleep is far better than a restless eight.

What to do

Research suggests that women with PCOS may be prone to sleep problems due to the hormonal fluctuations associated with the condition,[44] but there are things you can do to improve your chances of a good night's sleep.

Step one: boost your serotonin

Serotonin is a hormone that promotes good sleep. There are a number of ways you can boost levels in your body.

Eat foods that will boost your supply naturally. Serotonin is manufactured within your body from the amino acid tryptophan, found in many foods — notably soybeans, lean meat, fish, eggs and low-fat cheese and skimmed milk. That's why the old advice to drink a glass of warm milk before you sleep can work wonders.

In order for tryptophan to convert to serotonin it needs vitamin B_6, so you need to ensure that your diet is rich in B_6. You can get B_6 from foods such as spinach, fish, lentils, carrots and potatoes.

You should make sure you eat foods that are rich in minerals — especially calcium, magnesium (often called nature's own tranquillizer) and silicon, as they can induce a calming state of mind — while a deficiency has been shown to cause sleep problems. Try to include more mineral-rich foods such as watercress, broccoli, parsley, leeks, spinach, almonds, sesame seeds, sunflower seeds, dried figs, pulses, beans, lentils, brown rice, peaches, bananas, dates, avocados, raisins and sea vegetables in your diet.

You also need plenty of exposure to daylight. Light is necessary for serotonin production, so try to make sure that you spend some time outdoors every day. Even if it's an overcast day, your body will feel the benefits.

Step two: good sleeping habits

The next step is to establish some good sleeping habits. If you struggle to fall asleep, or wake in the middle of the night and then can't get back to sleep, there are some basic good sleep strategies that can help.

Wind down an hour or so before you go to bed and avoid exercise in the evening. Activity delays melatonin production (when night comes, serotonin converts to melatonin). Try having a warm bath, perhaps with relaxing aromatherapy oils such as lavender or bergamot, or do some relaxation techniques such as lying on your bed tensing and then relaxing muscles throughout the body part in turn. Or perhaps you'd prefer to do some gentle stretches, make love, write in your diary, have a gentle massage, drink some chamomile tea or sprinkle a few drops of calming essential lavender oil on your pillow – anything that makes you feel relaxed. If you can't sleep after lying down for more than half an hour, get up and do something monotonous like ironing or reading. Then, when you feel sleepy again, go back to bed.

It isn't a good idea to eat a heavy meal or drink a lot before bedtime. Your body needs to rest, not digest, so ideally eat no later than 8 p.m. Also avoid stimulants like caffeine and alcohol before bedtime.

Make sure your mattress and bed are comfortable. Use your bed for sleeping and sex only, so you only associate it with rest and pleasure. Block out noise and light (light will impair the production of melatonin). Sleep in a well-ventilated, cool (but not cold) room – around 60°F/15°C, as body temperature naturally falls at night.

Stick to a regular sleep/wake pattern, even at weekends. Ideally you should aim to be in bed for around 11 p.m. every night, as studies show that people who sleep before midnight awake more refreshed than those who go to bed in the small hours.

If you want to nap during the day, sleep expert Chris Idzikowski from the Surrey Sleep Research Centre suggests that 25 minutes just after lunch is the optimum time to beat fatigue and boost concentration. Any longer than that and you risk fragmented sleep at night.

An hour before you go to bed, write a 'to do' list and lay your clothes out for the next day so that you won't need to rush around in the morning. If you find it hard to switch off from the day's events, lie in bed and focus your mind on something that's relaxing and happy – your dream holiday or happy memories, perhaps – and you'll find it easier to let go of the day.

If you still find it hard to drop off, try not to let it get you down. The more you worry about not sleeping, the more stressed you're going to get. The chances are that if you sleep badly one night you'll sleep soundly the next, especially if you're eating healthily and exercising daily.

STRESS MANAGEMENT

66 *Whenever I have a deadline at work or some kind of personal crisis, my symptoms flare up. Friends say they can always tell when I'm upset or have had an argument with my boyfriend because my acne flares up. But it's not just my acne, if I'm feeling stressed I've noticed that my periods go haywire as well. What's going on?* 99

Anna, 25

If you find that your PCOS symptoms get worse when you're stressed or going through an emotionally testing time, you're not alone. Your emotional state has a powerful effect on your body, and here's why.

Adrenaline is the hormone most of us associate with stress. This is the hormone released in the well-known 'flight or fight' response, and it has a powerful effect on the body. When you feel threatened or sense danger, your heart speeds up and the arteries tighten to raise blood pressure. Your liver immediately releases emergency stores of glucose into your bloodstream to give you the energy to fight or escape. Your digestion and reproductive cycle slow down because they aren't necessary for immediate survival, and your blood's clotting ability increases to help prepare your body in the event of injury.

All this means that you're primed and ready to run, attack and react more quickly than normal. It happens very quickly, and ideally should last long enough to help you take action or get out of danger. This survival response worked well thousands of years ago when dangers such as a fierce animals threatened our survival, but the trouble is most modern-day stresses, such as missing the train or getting stuck in traffic can't always be resolved by action. You just sit there and seethe. And so, what was designed to be a short-term stress reaction can go on for long periods of time.

If you're under long-term stress, your adrenal glands become increasingly overworked and have difficulty producing hormones in the right amount. As well as too much adrenaline, too much cortisol and testosterone are released, and this can drive your body toward insulin resistance, weight gain, depression and irregular periods. Prolonged stress also affects your digestion so that you aren't getting the nutritional value from the foods you eat, and your immune system so that you're more susceptible to infections. Most importantly, your risk of high blood pressure and heart disease increases dramatically.

Stress-management is essential for women with PCOS, not just for their physical and emotional health but for the prevention of insulin resistance and diabetes,[45] high blood pressure,[46] heart disease[47] and possibly cancer (high levels of stress have been linked with an increased risk of cancer[48]).

If stress is a problem for you, you are not alone. Research suggests that women with PCOS often can't deal with stress effectively and have an increased response to stress due to the hormonal fluctuations associated with the condition.[49]

The following stress management tips can help:

- Learn to recognize when you are stressed. Many of us have got so used to living with stress, we don't even recognize the signs anymore. Common signals include irritability, lack of concentration, mood swings and fatigue and digestive problems.
- Deal with short-term stress, such as sitting in heavy traffic, with simple relaxation techniques such as tensing your muscles and relaxing them or deep breathing to a count of 10. Other techniques include stretching, talking with friends, drinking calming herbal teas like chamomile or lemon balm, having a good laugh, stroking your pet, day-dreaming about relaxing places you've been to or hugging someone you love.
- Research has shown that massage can help lower blood pressure, improve breathing, boost mood and well-being and aid circulation.[50] Some experts believe that massage helps the brain produce

endorphins, the chemicals that act as natural painkillers. The sense of well-being you get from a massage can lower the amount of stress hormones circulating in your body.

- Yoga is a great stress reducer. Studies suggest that it can help prevent hypertension and poor health. MIND, the UK's leading mental health charity, recommends yoga as the single most effective stress buster.[51]

- Meditation is a good way to deal with mental and physical stress. Scientists led by Vernon Barnes at the Medical College of Georgia studied transcendental meditation with 32 healthy adults and concluded that it can lower blood pressure. Other research suggests that it can also help prevent heart disease and cancer.[52]

- Don't waste energy trying to change what you can't. Try to identify those situations that trigger stress, and if you can't avoid them find ways to accept and manage them with a minimum amount of stress.

- Simply talking to friends, family and partners can ease stress. Dr Dean Ornish, Clinical Professor of Medicine and the University of California, San Francisco, in his pioneering text *Love and Survival: The Healing Power of Intimacy* has shown that loving relationships and support networks can all keep your blood pressure and your heart healthy. Remember, stress can make your symptoms worse and increase your risk of disease, so get yourself a support network. This could be your partner or family and friends, but if you don't feel you've anyone you can talk to, a trained counsellor can help you get in touch with your feelings and give you tips on how to deal with stress.

- Never forget that other women with PCOS can be a great support during bad times and good. PCOS support groups like Verity in the UK and PCOSupport in the US are excellent places to turn to (see Useful Contacts chapter, beginning on page 297).

- Set aside time to relax every day, no matter what. And try not to be a perfectionist. The housework can wait, the answerphone can take your calls and if the kids are screaming, put them to bed half an hour earlier so you can get some much-needed relaxation. Give yourself a break – you deserve it.

We know we've said this time and time again, but do make sure that you're eating a healthy diet and getting enough exercise. The adrenals rely on vitamin C, B, zinc and magnesium to make hormones and function well; these nutrients are rapidly decreased when you're under stress. If you're eating a healthy balanced diet with lots of fruits, vegetables and wholegrains, you should be getting all you need. A good multivitamin and -mineral every day as back-up also makes sense. As for exercise, just 20 minutes a day reduces stress levels, boosts your energy and balances your hormones. It also stimulates circulation, improves digestion and encourages your body to get rid of toxins.

Finally, try to have a more optimistic approach to life. According to Dr Candace Pert, Research Professor in the Department of Physiology and Biophysics at Georgetown University Medical Centre in Washington, DC, and author of *Molecules of Emotion: Why We Feel What We Feel*, emotions such as fear, panic, anxiety, jealousy and anger can trigger the stress response, affect your blood sugar levels and increase your likelihood of poor health and disease. In her own words, 'a healthy mind is a healthy body.' Research is still in its infancy, but increasingly both scientists and mind/body experts believe that grumpy, pessimistic, angry people are more likely to get heart disease and suffer from poor health than people who are more relaxed and upbeat.[53] The Protection Plan encourages you to take care of your body, but you mustn't overlook the importance of your emotions. Don't let a 'half-empty' attitude poison your life. Seek out the sunny and positive and open yourself up to the possibility that the glass just might be half-full.

66 *I'm convinced that stress is linked to my PCOS. I had a really bad relationship with my father. Don't want to go into the details but it was horrible. For years I tried to make sense of the past and fit the pieces of the puzzle together, and just before my father died we had a kind of reconciliation. The sense of relief I felt was huge and I remember going home and crying for three hours flat. Two weeks later I had my first period in 10 years, and they've been regular ever since. My other symptoms seemed to vanish, too, and I can't help but feel that there's a*

strong connection, as if the pain and hurt I was holding inside me was putting the brakes on my reproductive cycle. It was almost as if my body was saying, "Look, you need to sort this out before you can move forward with your life". **99**

Ingrid, 26

ONE STEP AT A TIME

Having read the Protection Plan guidelines in this chapter you'll be able to recognize where changes in your diet and lifestyle need to be made and how these changes can help you beat not just the symptoms of PCOS but the risk of potential long-term complications. Remember, though, to take one small step at a time and move forward gradually. All the changes recommended are designed to get right at the heart of the underlying hormonal imbalances that cause PCOS and the complications associated with it, rather than offering quick-fix solutions. Healthy living and eating are positive changes to last you a lifetime.

Small and gradual change is the best way to create long-term improvement in your health and well-being. It can be tough when you don't see immediate results, but the advantage of taking things slowly is that you tend to get long-lasting results. Think of it as if it were a savings plan – if you look after the little things (in this case the daily activities that can help you avoid acne or going up a dress size), then the big things (the risk of hypertension, heart disease, diabetes and cancer) will look after themselves. Taking charge of your health and taking things one step at a time will help you improve your health and well-being now and in the years to come.

REFERENCES

1.   Harber, B. J. *et al.*, 'Energy balance and reproductive function in active women', *Can J Appl Physiol* 2004 Feb; 29 (1): 48–58

2. Norman, N. J. *et al.*, 'Improving reproductive performance in overweight/obese women with effective weight management', *Hum Reprod Update* 2004 May-Jun; 10 (3): 267–80

3. Koukouvov, G. *et al.*, 'Quality of life, psychological and physiological changes following exercise training in patients with chronic heart failure', *J Rehabil Med* 2004 Jan; 36 (1): 36–41

4. Charkoudian, N. *et al.*, 'Physiologic considerations for exercise performance in women', *Clin Chest Med* 2004 Jun; 25 (2): 247–55

5. Ross, R. *et al.*, 'Exercise-induced reduction in obesity and insulin resistance in women: a randomized controlled trial', *Obes Res* 2004 May; 12 (5): 789–98

6. Tsai, J. C. *et al.*, 'The beneficial effect of regular endurance exercise training on blood pressure and quality of life in patients with hypertension', *Clin Exp Hypertens* 2004 Apr; 26 (3): 255–65

7. Wagh, D. *et al.*, 'Treatment of metabolic syndrome', *Expert Rev Cardiovasc Ther* 2004 Mar; 2 (2): 213–28

8. Enger, S. M. *et al.*, 'Exercise activity, body size and premenopausal breast cancer survival', *Br J Cancer* 2004 Jun 1; 90 (11): 2138–41

9. McClung, B. L. *et al.*, 'Reducing your risk of osteoporosis', *Nurs Manage* 2001 Apr; Suppl: 4–5, 8

10. Rahman, T. *et al.*, 'The Purpose in Life and Academic Behaviour of Problem Students in Bangladesh', *Social Indicators Research* 1996; 39 (1): 59–64

11. Henning, B. F. *et al.*, 'Vitamin supplementation during weight reduction – favourable effect on homocysteine metabolism', *Res Exp Med* (Berl) 1998 Jul; 198 (1): 37–42

12. Evans, G. W. *et al.*, 'Composition and biological activity of chromium-pyridine carboxylate complexes', *J Inorg Biochem* 1993; 49: 177–87

13. American Diabetics Association, 'Magnesium supplementation in the treatment of diabetes', *Diabetes Care* 1992; 15: 1065–7

14. Van Gall, L. *et al.*, 'Biochemical and clinical aspects of co-enzyme Q10', *Journal of Vitaminology* 1984; 4: 369

15. Chasens, E. R. *et al.*, 'Insulin resistance and obstructive sleep apnea: is increased sympathetic stimulation the link?', *Biol Res Nurs* 2003 Oct; 5 (2): 87–96

16. Larkin, A., 'Linkage of serum leptin levels in families with sleep apnea', *Int J Obes Relat Metab Disord* advance online publications 2004 Dec 21; doi: 10.1038/sj.ijo.0802872

17. www.reuters.co.uk/newsPackag ... =topNews&storyID=561238§ion=news

18. Tremblay, A. *et al.*, 'Obesity: a disease or a biological adaption?' *Obes Rev* 2000 May; 1 (1): 27–35

19. Singleton, D. W. *et al.*, 'Xenoestrogen exposure and mechanisms of endocrine

disruption', *Front Biosci* 2003 Jan 1; 8: s110–8; Ibaretta, D. *et al.*, 'Possible health impact of phytoestrogens and xenoestrogens in food', *APMIS* 2001 Mar; 109 (3): 161–84

20. Recchia, A. *et al.*, 'Xenoestrogens and the induction of proliferative effects in breast cancer cells via direct activation of oestrogen receptor alpha', *Food Addit Contam* 2004 Feb; 21 (2): 134–44

21. Van Duyn, M. A. *et al.*, 'Overview of the health benefits of fruit and vegetable consumption for the dietetics professional: selected literature', *J Am Diet Assoc* 2000 Dec; 100 (12): 1511–21; Keck, A. S. *et al.*, 'Cruciferous vegetables: cancer protective mechanisms of glucosinolate hydrolysis products and selenium', *Integr Cancer Ther* 2004 Mar; 3 (1): 5–12

22. Krauze-Brzosko, K. *et al.*, 'Soy's phytoestrogens and their implication for human health', *Pol Merkuriusz Lek* 2002 Dec; 13 (78): 526–9

23. Tanasescu, M. *et al.*, 'Dietary fat and cholesterol and the risk of cardiovascular disease among women with type 2 diabetes', *Am J Clin Nutr* 2004 Jun; 79 (6): 999–1005; Read, A. *et al.*, 'A primary care intervention programme for obesity and coronary heart disease risk factor reduction', *Br J Gen Pract* 2004 Apr; 54 (501): 272–8

24. Kruger, C. L. *et al.*, 'Safety evaluation of functional ingredients', *Food Chem Toxicol* 2003 Jun; 41 (6): 793–805

25. Renwick, R. W. *et al.*, 'Risk characterisation of chemicals in food and diet', *Food Chem Toxicol* 2003 Sep; 41 (9): 1211–71; Denner, W. H. *et al.*, 'Colourings and preservatives in food', *Hum Nutr Appl Nutr* 1984 Dec; 38 (6): 435–49

26. Johnston, K. L. *et al.*, 'Coffee acutely modifies gastrointestinal hormone secretion and glucose tolerance in humans: glycemic effects of chlorogenic acid and caffeine', *Am J Clin Nutr* 2003 Oct; 78 (4): 728–33

27. Kurtis, J. M. *et al.*, 'Effects of cigarette smoking, caffeine consumption, and alcohol intake on fecundability', *Am J Epidemiol* 1997 Jul 1; 146 (1): 32–41

28. Gronbaek, M. *et al.*, 'Changes in alcohol intake and mortality: a longitudinal population-based study', *Epidemiology* 2004 Mar; 15 (2): 222–8

29. Kroenke, C. H. *et al.*, 'A cross-sectional study of alcohol consumption patterns and biologic markers of glycemic control among 459 women', *Diabetes Care* 2003 Jul; 26 (7): 1971

30. Coombes, R. *et al.*, 'One hospitality worker a week dies from passive smoking, study shows', *BMJ* 2004 May 22; 328 (7450): 1222

31. Davis, R. M. *et al.*, 'Exposure to environmental tobacco smoke: identifying and protecting those at risk', *JAMA* 1998 Dec 9; 280 (22): 1947–49

32. Henley, S. J. *et al.*, 'Association between exclusive pipe smoking and mortality from cancer and other diseases', *J Natl Cancer Inst* 2004 Jun 2; 96 (11): 853–61

33. Surendran, A. *et al.*, 'Studies linking breast cancer to deodorants smell rotten, experts say', *Nat Med* 2004 Mar; 10 (3): 216

34. Melish, M. E. *et al.*, 'Vaginal tampon model for toxic shock syndrome', *Rev Infect Dis* 1989 Jan-Feb; 11 Suppl 1: S238–46 (discussion pages S246–7)

35. Bryant, M. A. *et al.*, 'Sick and tired: does sleep have a vital role in the immune system?', *Nat Rev Immunol* 2004 Jun; 4 (6): 457–67

36. Everson, C. A. *et al.*, 'Reductions in circulating anabolic hormones induced by sustained sleep deprivation in rats', *Am J Physiol Endocrinol Metab* 2004 Jun; 286 (6): E1060–70

37. Chasens, E. R. *et al.*, 'Insulin resistance and obstructive sleep apnea: is increased sympathetic stimulation the link?', *Biol Res Nurs* 2003 Oct; 5 (2): 87–96; Vigg, A. *et al.*, 'Sleep in Type 2 diabetes', *J Assoc Physicians India* 2003 May; 51: 479–81

38. Coughlin, S. R. *et al.*, 'Obstructive sleep apnoea is independently associated with an increased prevalence of metabolic syndrome', *Eur Heart J* 2004 May; 25 (9): 735–41

39. Li, A. M. *et al.*, 'Obstructive sleep apnoea and obesity', *Hong Kong Med J* 2004 Apr; 10 (2): 144

40. Sharabi, Y. *et al.*, 'Sleep apnea as a risk factor for hypertension', *Curr Opin Nephrol Hypertens* 2004 May; 13 (3): 359–64; Goodfriend, T. L. *et al.*, 'Resistant hypertension, obesity, sleep apnea, and aldosterone: theory and therapy', *Hypertension* 2004 Mar; 43 (3): 518–24

41. Meritt, S. L. *et al.*, 'Sleep-disordered breathing and the association with cardiovascular risk', *Prog Cardiovasc Nurs* 2004 Winter; 19 (1): 19–27

42. Fortner, B. V. *et al.*, 'Sleep and quality of life in breast cancer patients', *J Pain Symptom Manage* 2002 Nov; 24 (5): 471–80

43. Patel, S. R., 'A prospective study of sleep duration and mortality risk in women', *Sleep* 2004 May 1; 27 (3): 440–4: 'STUDY OBJECTIVES: It is commonly believed that 8 hours of sleep per night is optimal for good health. However, recent studies suggest the risk of death is lower in those sleeping 7 hours. Our results confirm previous findings that mortality risk in women is lowest among those sleeping 6 to 7 hours. Further research is needed to understand the mechanisms by which short and long sleep times can affect health.'

44. Sanders, M. H. *et al.*, 'Increased risk of obstructive sleep apnea in obese women with polycystic ovary syndrome (a review of two related articles). Articles reviewed: "Increased prevalence of obstructive sleep apnea syndrome in obese women with polycystic ovary syndrome" and "Polycystic ovary syndrome is associated with obstructive sleep apnea and daytime sleepiness: role of insulin resistance"', *Sleep Med* 2002 May; 3 (3): 287–9

45. Grey, M. *et al.*, 'Preliminary testing of a program to prevent type 2 diabetes

among high-risk youth', *J Sch Health* 2004 Jan; 74 (1): 10–15; Legro, R. S. *et al.*, 'Detecting insulin resistance in polycystic ovary syndrome: purposes and pitfalls', *Obstet Gynecol Surv* 2004 Feb; 59 (2): 141–54

46. McCraty, R. *et al.*, 'Impact of a workplace stress reduction program on blood pressure and emotional health in hypertensive employees', *J Altern Complement Med* 2003 Jun; 9 (3): 355–69

47. Haskell, L. W. *et al.*, 'Cardiovascular disease prevention and lifestyle interventions: effectiveness and efficacy', *J Cardiovasc Nurs* 2003 Sep-Oct; 18 (4): 245–55

48. Murr, C. *et al.*, 'Re: Personality and the risk of cancer', *J Natl Cancer Inst* 2003 Nov 5; 95 (21): 1638

49. Coffey, S. *et al.*, 'The effect of polycystic ovary syndrome on health-related quality of life', *Gynecol Endocrinol* 2003 Oct; 17 (5): 379–86

50. Soden, K. *et al.*, 'A randomized controlled trial of aromatherapy massage in a hospice setting', *Palliat Med* 2004 Mar; 18 (2): 87–92

51. Sianani, G. *et al.*, 'Non-drug therapy in prevention and control of hypertension', *J Assoc Physicians India* 2003 Oct; 51: 1001–6

52. Tacon, A. M. *et al.*, 'Mindfulness meditation, anxiety reduction, and heart disease: a pilot study', *Fam Community Health* 2003 Jan-Mar; 26 (1): 25–33; Speca, M. *et al.*, 'A randomized, wait-list controlled clinical trial: the effect of a mindfulness meditation-based stress reduction program on mood and symptoms of stress in cancer outpatients', *Psychosom Med* 2000 Sep-Oct; 62 (5): 613–22

53. Pitkala, L. H. *et al.*, 'Positive life orientation as a predictor of 10-year outcome in an aged population', *J Clin Epidemiol* 2004 Apr; 57 (4): 409–14

Part Three
Success

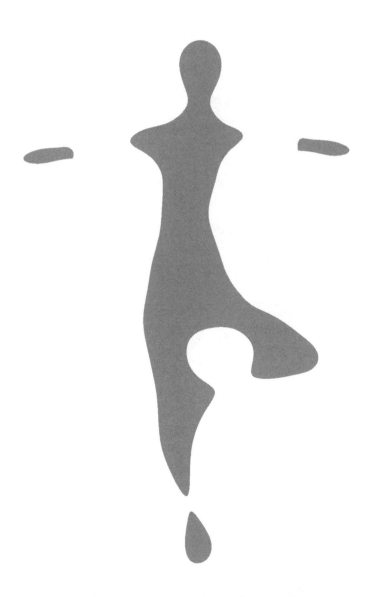

13 Staying on Track

The Protection Plan is something you can do yourself – but sometimes it can be hard. This section of the book is devoted to combating the bad habits and difficult situations that can keep you from progressing: lack of motivation, unwillingness to face up to the facts, comfort-eating, eating disorders, fatigue, addiction to sugar, and the day-to-day pressures of life.

LACK OF MOTIVATION

66 I'm great at starting things but not so good at finishing them or even getting half way. I've got PCOS and I know I feel better when I eat healthily and exercise regularly, and for a couple of weeks I do well, but then I get bored and start missing workouts or eating fatty foods again. I don't do it consciously. Before I know it I'm back to my old habits. I'd love to be able to break this pattern. 99

Susi, 21

Working to keep your symptoms and the long-term health risks at bay is a day-in, day-out project for the long haul. So how do you maintain your new healthy behaviours and stay motivated? You find ways to adapt to the change.

We've all had big changes in our lives that instantly make everything different, like moving house, changing jobs, getting married, having a child or adopting a pet. At times these changes can seem overwhelming, but after a while you learn to adapt and, once you have, you often can't imagine how you got on before you had a child or moved house. It's exactly the same for changes in your lifestyle. Once you start to create new habits there will come a time when you'll look back and find it hard to imagine life without them. Old habits start to feel uncomfortable. Missing your workouts or eating fatty foods, for example, will feel strange to you because they will no longer be part of who you are. Another example is putting sugar in your tea: once you've gone without for a while, tea with sugar will taste sickly and unpleasant to you.

If you do find yourself at the point when old habits don't feel comfortable, congratulations! You're ready to move from changing habits to maintaining them. Perhaps surprisingly, though, it's when you're at this point, so close to success, that you're actually at your most vulnerable. It's easy to get motivated about the active change phase; the trouble can start once the changes become, in themselves, your new routine. So how can you stick with it?

Plan ahead, monitor, take action if necessary and keep your focus.

Maintaining lifestyle habits to prevent the risk of diabetes, high blood pressure, obesity and heart disease is in some ways the same as what big corporations call *continuous quality improvement*. This involves planning and then carrying out your plans. It also involves checking your progress and acting to make improvements where necessary.

For example, you may plan to exercise more, and may even have begun doing so. It's important, though, also to have a monitoring process in place for times when you slip back into your old habits. A good way to do this is to implement some basic checks. By periodically recording your weight, exercise and eating habits, for example, you can gauge how you're doing. You'll see how much progress you're making and also will be able to work out the steps you need to take to get back on (or stay on) track.

Self-monitoring in this way can involve recording your weight, stress levels, eating and exercise habits in a journal or notebook or daily planner. Perhaps you want to see how well you're doing with your fat grams or your sugar intake, so you record what you're eating, in what portions, and how much fat and sugar it contains. Are you getting enough exercise? Try recording your daily activities to see if it all adds up.

Self-monitoring can be extremely motivating. It can help you stay on track when the going gets tough by reminding you that you're the one in charge of your health, just as a corporation is in charge of its work flow, services and programs. A good CEO will continually monitor quality control. The key to your success on the Protection Plan is to continue checking how you're doing, and acting, whenever you feel you're slipping.

Everything we suggest on the Protection Plan will add to your success, but motivation is key. Self-monitoring is one way to help you stay focused for the long haul, but there are many others. Learning how others have kept their focus can be helpful. Take Debbie, for example.

Debbie was diagnosed with PCOS in her late twenties. When she learned about the increased risk of diabetes, she knew she had to take action as her father had diabetes, her aunt died from the complications of diabetes and her brother had recently been diagnosed. So when her doctor said she was insulin resistant she wasn't surprised. Her doctor told her that to prevent diabetes she needed to eat healthy food and exercise. Since that day, Debbie has worked hard to make nutritious food choices and exercise four or five times a week. Her insulin levels have returned to the normal range and she plans to keep them that way. She wants to live a long life to avoid the complications of PCOS.

The lesson to learn from Debbie is that even though PCOS and a strong family background of diabetes dramatically increased her chances of developing diabetes herself, she has reduced her odds and changed the outcome. She isn't letting nature take its course.

Amanda is also working to prevent the complications of PCOS. When she was pregnant her blood pressure went sky high and she had to have six weeks of bed rest. After her baby was born, Amanda's blood pressure normalized but she knew that, with PCOS, she had a higher than normal risk of getting high blood pressure. How does she stay motivated? She focuses on how good she feels when she eats and lives healthily, when she gets good quality sleep and regular exercise. Debbie notices the short-term benefits and they help her stay focused on her long-term goal – PCOS protection.

Sarah keeps her motivation going with a combination of positive thinking and visualization techniques. After several unsuccessful attempts at healthy eating and regular exercise, she bought a life-coaching book and began to see that she was, in fact, programming herself to fail. She was telling herself that she had no self-control and was lazy and fat, and the subconscious part of her mind – which always does what it's told – was living up (or down!) to her expectations. She decided to try using positive descriptions of herself – such as healthy, vibrant, attractive, confidant and so on – instead. Sarah made a point of concentrating on positive images and thoughts about herself every day, and if she found herself using negative 'self-talk' she replaced it with the positive kind. She realized the importance of aligning her thoughts and actions to her healthy eating and living goals. Instead of blaming others or telling herself she was weak willed or that she could not do it, she took responsibility and told herself she could – and even when she wasn't entirely convinced, it worked a treat!

Sarah also learned to envision herself achieving her goals in the future and to see herself as the person she wanted to be. She would imagine scenes, such as running after her grandchildren on the beach 20 years hence. Sarah finds self-empowering, positive-thinking techniques like these help her stay on track with her lifestyle changes. She thinks of herself as her own winning coach.

Debbie, Amanda and Sarah all found different ways to keep their motivation going and take charge of their health. We can all learn a lot from them. You need to find what works best for you, but whatever it is, the bottom line is always to keep your eyes on the prize: lowering your risk of the complications associated with PCOS. Remembering why you're doing what you're doing and focusing on the health benefits of your actions both now and in the future can keep you motivated for a long and happy life.

HEAD IN THE SAND

❝ *Yes, I've got PCOS, but most of the time I feel OK. I can't get my head around the idea that I might be at increased risk of really serious conditions such as diabetes, just because I get the odd bout of acne and have — like millions of other women — irregular periods.* **❞**

Nadia, 25

You may find that even though you know and understand the changes you need to make, you just can't bring yourself to make them. You stick your head in the sand and tell yourself that the future is a long way off and, besides, it couldn't possibly happen to you.

Most of us are afraid of change and keep putting it off. Life needs to get pretty rough or painful for us to change, and many people only begin to drop old habits when the discomfort starts to outweigh the benefits. For example, many people only give up smoking when they have a heart attack, even though they have known for years that smoking increases their risk.

Many women with PCOS can only find the strength to change after something unpleasant makes them face up to reality. Did your doctor (or this book) warn you of the increased risks of PCOS? Did a recent episode of dizziness or mood swings make you realize that your insulin resistance could be edging you slowly towards full-blown diabetes? Has a recent photo of yourself made you feel sad? Have you found yourself crying in the changing room while trying on new clothes? Instead of trying to downplay or ignore these triggers because of the discomfort and pain they cause, you should take them on as a powerful driving force to propel you toward change.

EATING YOUR FEELINGS

❝ *If I feel sad, disappointed, guilty, scared or angry or my PCOS symptoms get worse, my first response is always to reach for food — preferably* *chocolate. I know it isn't good for me and it's going to make my symptoms worse, but I've done this for so long now I don't know any other way of coping. I wish there were a way out for me, as more often than not these days I feel ashamed and sad after a bout of comfort eating, like I'm letting myself down.* 99

Monica, 31

Women and food have a complex relationship, regardless of whether or not they have PCOS. How many women do you know who don't worry about what they eat and what they weigh? There are loads of reasons for our troubled relationships with food, and PCOS only magnifies the problem – not just because of the body-image insecurities often associated with the condition, but because food and weight management are integral parts of any treatment plan.

If you're prone to comfort eating, it will be very hard for you to stick to the Protection Plan. That's why we urge you to work on healing your emotional relationship with food *before* you start. If you don't, you're putting yourself under too much pressure and just setting yourself up for disappointment.

Comfort eating is one of the biggest causes of weight gain in women, and it's particularly unhelpful if you've PCOS – we've seen how excess weight can trigger symptoms. If you do find yourself turning to food for comfort on a regular basis or think your difficult relationship with food is making it hard for you to stick to the plan, it's vital that you understand the link between food and mood so that you can move toward a healthier attitude to eating.

There's a reason why the comfort-eating foods of choice are often sugary and fatty. Within your brain, chemicals help transmit messages from one nerve cell to another. These chemicals – serotonin and norepinephrine (also called endorphins) affect the way you feel. Your body makes these endorphins from the food you eat, and the main sources of endorphins are sugary, carbohydrate-rich foods like white bread, cakes, chocolate and pasta. Trouble is, if you've got PCOS and you comfort eat with high-sugar foods, you'll end up not just with an endorphin rush but also with a surge of insulin, which is just what you need to avoid.

It's not just stress or anxiety that can make you comfort-eat; any kind of nutritional deficiency can make you eat more sugary foods to try and boost your energy levels, setting up a vicious cycle of nutritional deficiency and depression.

A healthy relationship with food is yet another key to success on the Protection Plan. Food is a powerful tool you can use to improve your physical health, protect yourself against disease and boost your emotional health. You're eating not just to improve symptoms and your chances of good health in the future, but to feel happier and more content.

So if comfort eating is ruining your chances of success, what should you do?

First of all, *before* making any dietary changes, get your relationship with food on track. If your comfort eating is triggered by a PCOS-related problem such as acne, infertility or weight gain, ask your doctor to refer you to a counsellor who can help you with these issues. If you don't think your comfort eating is PCOS-related but caused by something else, you may want to see a counsellor who is a specialist in, say, building self-esteem, stress at work, coping with violence, relationship problems and so on. You may also find these 'building a healthy relationship with food' tips helpful:

- Food is not your enemy. If you 'ban' certain foods, such as chocolate, these are precisely the ones you'll crave. Guilt and food do not mix. Pete Cohen from *Lighten Up* points out that there's no such thing as an unhealthy food, only unhealthy attitudes toward food. For example, foods like chocolate and red meat are only unhealthy if you eat them in large amounts. If you enjoy them now and again, they won't do you any harm. If you can change your attitude to food you can eat healthily without feeling deprived and allow yourself the occasional indulgence without feeling guilty.

- Relax. If thinking about food makes you anxious, find other ways to ease the tension rather than reaching for the fridge door. Deep slow breaths, gently clenching and relaxing your muscles, phoning a friend, going for a walk, meditating or simply listening to your favourite music are just some of the many tried-and-tested ways to clear your mind and ease tension.

- Wait 20 minutes after you eat a meal or snack before eating more. It takes at least this amount of time for your brain to register that your stomach is full.

- If you really can't resist a food, take three bites of it. The first bite is heavenly bliss – really taste and enjoy it, let the food linger in your mouth. Thoroughly enjoy the second bite, too. Let the third bite emotionally register that you have had the food, then stop, letting go of any feelings of resentment and punishment that you might have had if you denied yourself it.

- When you do eat, focus on your food. Turn off the TV and don't read when you eat. Sit down to eat and put your knife and fork down between each mouthful so you can savour and enjoy your food properly. Make eating a memorable occasion.

- Reach for a glass of water if you're fighting the urge to snack. We often mistake thirst for hunger, as the trigger centres are very close to one another in the brain.

- A food-and-mood diary can help you to understand your eating habits. If comfort-eating has become a regular thing for you, you may have lost the ability to judge when you're really hungry.

- The next time you want to eat, ask yourself if you're really hungry. If you aren't sure, you probably aren't.

- You may think that you're treating yourself when you comfort eat but if it leads to weight gain and a worsening of your symptoms is that really a treat?

If you do comfort eat on a regular basis, your self-esteem could be fairly low and this will have a negative impact on eating habits. The first thing you need to understand is that you're an OK person and you deserve the best, and that includes eating the best. Positive statements you repeat to yourself over and over again until they sink in, such as 'I feel confident' or 'I can do this,' can help. Remind yourself, too, that you've a right to be assertive, to express your opinions and emotions and be the unique individual you are. Just because you've got PCOS doesn't make you any less of a woman. You also have the right to make mistakes and change your mind. There will be times when you eat things that aren't good for you. It's not a big deal. You can get back on track tomorrow.

Other self-esteem building tips include giving yourself lots of non-food treats, especially when things are stressful, such as a soothing massage, a new haircut or outfit, a trip to the theatre, curling up with a good book, giving yourself quality time to chill out and enjoy your own company, getting support from loved ones and people who make you feel good about yourself and, last but by no means least, being yourself and making sure your goals are what you, not what your partner, your family or your friends, want.

Many things about PCOS are uncertain, but one thing isn't: a healthy diet can improve your symptoms, protect your future health, increase the power of any medication you're on and help you enjoy your life. Remind yourself of this several times a day; write it down and stick it on your mirror, your desk, your fridge, even on your biscuit tin. If the going gets tough, you'll be reminded that by taking charge of your eating and making positive food choices you're doing all you can to improve your symptoms and protect your health in the future.

DISORDERED EATING

If you feel unhappy about the way you look and feel there's a risk you may go about trying to change this in the wrong way by starving yourself or bingeing on massive amounts of food and then vomiting or using laxatives to cleanse yourself, then you will know that you could be on your way to developing an eating disorder.

Any eating pattern or exercise routine that's taken to the extreme is dangerous. Your body does not get the nutrients it needs to maintain a healthy menstrual cycle, bingeing and starving trigger insulin resistance and the hormonal havoc this causes can make your symptoms worse and increase your long-term health risks.

Experts differ as to whether there's a link between PCOS and eating disorders. Some studies have suggested that as many as 60 per cent of women with eating problems may have also have PCOS,[1] though other research dismisses the link.[2] Since many women with PCOS have problems losing weight, a link wouldn't be surprising. Eating disorders are, however, such a complex and dangerous health concern that they are outside the scope of this book.[3] Needless to say, it's vital if you suspect that you've got an eating disorder that you ask your doctor for help and advice.

You may not think about food all the time or have a full-blown eating disorder like anorexia and bulimia, but you may feel you have an unhealthy or unhelpful attitude toward food or think about it more than is considered normal. Perhaps you're constantly dieting or switching from one exercise fad to another. If this is the case, in the long run it's just as damaging to your future health as a more obvious eating disorder. You won't be getting the nutrients you need to balance your hormones and your blood sugar, and this will make your symptoms worse. You'll also be increasing your risk of diabetes, heart disease, infertility and obesity. And weight loss will be harder because unhealthy eating confuses your metabolic rate so that when you do eat your body stores a greater proportion of what you eat as fat.

If you've got PCOS and start to binge, fast or yo-yo diet, not only will this make it impossible for you to stick to the plan, it will create nutritional deficiencies, trigger insulin problems and make your symptoms worse. If you feel that your eating patterns are spiralling out of control and the quality of your life is being affected, the advice and information in this book can certainly help, but it's crucial that you seek the support of your doctor, a dietician or a qualified nutritionist immediately.

JUST TOO TIRED

66I get up in the morning feeling like I need a good night's sleep. I've got PCOS and am insulin resistant and my doctor says that this could be making me feel more tired than usual, but there has to be something I can do. I'm scared I may have an accident or something, as recently I've been dozing off in the middle of the day. **99**

Chloe, 42

Fatigue isn't recognized as a symptom of PCOS, but many women with PCOS say they feel tired and low a lot of the time, and research backs this up.[4] When you're feeling run down it can be extra tough to keep to your healthy eating and lifestyle plan. Not only are you more tempted to take the easy option and grab processed convenience foods with little or no nutritional value but you're also more likely to reach for foods that give you a short-lived energy boost while making your symptoms worse. If fatigue is making it hard for you to keep going, the following recommendations may help:

- Get your blood sugar and hormones balanced – the Protection Plan diet guidelines can help.
- Avoid energy-sappers: sugar, alcohol, saturated fats, caffeine, white flour products and highly processed foods. Pesticides, hormones and additives also rob food of its energy potential.
- Make sure you drink enough water throughout the day.
- Get more energy-rich B-vitamin foods: wholegrains such as millet, buckwheat, rye and quinoa, corn, alfalfa and barley. If these grains are sprouted their energy quotient is increased many times. Fresh, green leafy vegetables are also rich in vitamin B.
- Protein, protein, protein: make sure your diet consists of 20 to 25 per cent good-quality low-fat protein and don't eat a carbohydrate snack unless it's combined with some form of protein.
- Fatigue can be caused by iron-deficiency anaemia. See your doctor for a blood test to check your iron levels. Replace drinking black tea with herbal alternatives (tea contains tannin, which can leach

away iron supplies), eat iron-rich wholegrains and wheat germ, and get lots of vitamin C-rich green leafy vegetables. Also allow yourself a small portion of red meat now and again; if you're a vegetarian, make sure your soya milk and cereals are iron fortified and you snack on iron-rich apricots or a small bar of dark chocolate.

- Other essential energy-producing nutrients: magnesium (found in green vegetables, nuts and seeds), copper (found in oats, salmon and mushrooms), co-enzyme Q10 (found in spinach, beef and peanuts), essential fatty acids (found in flax seeds and hempseeds)
- Eat more raw foods. For sustained energy throughout the day experiment, with a variety of raw fruit and vegetable juices – in salads, with hummus as a snack, grated on a sandwich.
- Sunflower oil and sunflower seeds are packed with essential fatty acids, vitamins, minerals and protein. They are a fine energy pick-me-up, especially when combined with some dried fruit.
- Sea vegetables or seaweed are a highly digestible source of minerals. They can improve digestion and enhance mental energy. Wild blue-green algae contains virtually every nutrient known to man and can provide a feeling of well-being and vitality.
- As we've already seen, as well as a healthy diet, getting a good night's sleep, exercising regularly and losing weight (if you're overweight) will not only keep your symptoms at bay but also be a great vitality booster. But there are other less well-known ways to boost your energy levels and fight fatigue; one of the most enjoyable is to laugh more. Keep your sense of humour well stimulated, spend time with people who make you feel happy, watch comedies on TV or the stage, dance to upbeat music – whatever makes you smile.
- It also helps to keep your creative powers well stimulated. Are you passionate about something? When you're focused and motivated, you feel alert and energized. Play thinking games, read a good book, take up a new interest or hobby, learn a new language, join a debating society, enrol in an evening class – anything that can help keep your mind stimulated and fully awake.

- Lime essential oil, lemon or peppermint in your morning bath can be invigorating, and a cup or peppermint, lemon or ginger is a great alternative pick-me-up to coffee or tea.
- There are also a number of therapies you might like to experiment with that are thought to boost energy, such as yoga, tai chi, massage, aromatherapy and acupuncture.
- Finally, have you ever noticed how great you feel when it's a beautiful sunny day outside? You feel eager to go out and live. Then think about how you feel in the winter time – it's cold and dark and you want to stay in bed. This is because when you're exposed to sunlight not only do you get a top-up of energy-boosting vitamin D but your body starts to produce serotonin, which makes you feel alert and happy. So, light up your life. You could buy special bright white light bulbs but, better still, get out in the daylight and the fresh air for at least 20 minutes a day.
- Bear in mind that thyroid problems, anaemia (lack of iron), nutritional deficiencies, allergies, food intolerance and infection can all lower your energy levels, so check with your doctor to rule these out. It's also well known that fatigue is linked to emotional factors like depression. When you feel low, fatigue can take over. Wanting to stay in bed and sleep a lot is a sign of depression; if you think this might have something to do with your tiredness, do see your doctor.

ADDICTION TO SUGAR

66*I have a sweet tooth. If I pass a vending machine or a sweet shop I find it impossible to resist. I have to buy something. I'm no better at home. I can't drink tea or coffee without lashings of sugar, and if there are sweets or biscuits in the house I have to eat them. I once tore open some chocolates that were a gift for my mum. I'd like to eat healthily, as I do believe it will ease my PCOS and make me feel better, but sugar is my downfall. I can't live without it.*99

Rachel, 24

You may find that you're so addicted to sugar it's hard for you to keep to the Protection Plan guidelines. Your brain relies solely on glucose for thinking and functioning, and when blood sugar (glucose) levels fall too low, the brain suffers and demands immediate sugar for relief. That's why you get an uncontrollable urge to reach for a chocolate bar. There's no such thing as will power when your brain is sending strong signals that it needs sugar to rescue it from low glucose levels. Your satisfying the craving causes a surge of glucose, followed by an insulin release, but for every insulin surge there's a drop in blood sugar. This wild roller-coaster ride never ends.

If you do find the sugar habit hard to break, the best remedy is to make sure you eat enough protein and good fat according to the Protection Plan diet guidelines. Protein and fat, you may recall, slow down the release of sugar into your bloodstream. It's also important to eat little and often, to keep your blood sugar levels steady, and to keep an eye on the glycaemic index when making your food choices. Taking chromium supplements may also help control sugar cravings. Researchers have found that many people with insulin resistance and diabetes have a chromium deficiency. The organic, chelated forms such as chromium polynicotinate and chromium picolinate have been found to be the most potent and easiest for the body to absorb. See also our tips for avoiding sugar and dealing with food cravings on pages 75–77 and 184.

TOO MUCH STRESS, TOO LITTLE TIME

'I've read the Protection Plan guidelines and it all makes perfect sense to me and I'm sure it would help me feel better and reduce my long-term health risks. Trouble is I just don't have the time to think about what I eat and fit exercise into my schedule. I'm a working mum with three kids — how can I find time for me? **99**

Marion, 40

It's often during times of stress or pressure that resolve weakens and it's hard to stick to the Protection Plan guidelines. Not only are you more likely to reach for comfort foods, you simply haven't got time to think about what's the healthiest option. If your life is stressful or you're going through a period of stress, there are ways to stress-proof your diet.

Plan ahead

Draw up a daily eating and exercise schedule, so you know what you're going to eat for your snacks and main meals and when you're going to take your exercise. Without forward planning you're more likely to skimp on your exercise and make yourself vulnerable to overeating, especially at the most trying time for comfort eaters (3 p.m. to midnight). 'What, more planning?' you may say – 'Haven't I got enough stress already?' But knowing what you're going to eat and how you're going to plan your day will limit uncertainty and guilt, and make things easier and less stressful in the long run.

Dining out

If you need to dine out, don't panic, just pay attention to what you're ordering. If you make healthy food choices on the menu, stay away from the bread basket, drink lots of water instead of fizzy or alcoholic drinks, go for lots of soup and salad, tomato- or wine-based sauces rather than cheesy, buttery ones, and ask for dressings on the side, you should be fine. When it comes to dessert, go for fruit or try the 'three bites' technique we suggested earlier.

Healthy snacks to the rescue!

Keep lots of healthy snacks to hand, in your fridge, car or desk so they are there when you need them and you don't have to rush to the chocolate machine.

Remember breakfast

Never skip breakfast. This will just make you eat too much later in the day. Make sure, too, that you have a mid-morning snack about three hours after breakfast – ideally some protein, like yoghurt and a piece of fruit. Eat your mid-afternoon snack about three hours after lunch. This should include protein and carbohydrate and be low in fat – for example soup with crackers, cottage cheese and fruit and so on. And finally, try to eat most of your daily calories before 5 p.m., and don't eat too much after 8 p.m.

Cravings

If you really, really crave a sweet food, treat yourself to it now and again. The occasional chocolate bar, slice of white bread, piece of cake or glass of wine won't hurt you. Go ahead and really enjoy every mouthful – remember the 80/20 rule. Just don't get into the habit of turning to alcohol (which is very high in sugar) or other sugary foods and drinks as a way to relax. The same applies to cooking: don't beat yourself up if once in a while you have a ready-prepared meal, if cooking would make you tired and stressed.

Keep cooking simple

Many comforting dishes are actually easy to prepare. Soup with beans, for example, or baked apples with raisins or low-fat cheese on toast – all simple but delicious and nutritious. Eating should be a source of pleasure. The last thing you want to do is make it a source of stress.

Be prepared

Sometimes however much we plan ahead, things change and eating routines have to adapt quickly. Keep your cupboards, fridge and freezer well stocked with emergency healthy foods such as soup, beans, tinned vegetables and low-fat frozen meals. Chopped fresh fruits and vegetables make great sandwich fillers and are good to nibble on when you feel hungry. If your routine is totally disrupted, for example the kitchen floods or you're moving house, keep as active as you can and help yourself to fruit, vegetables and wholegrain bread sandwiches rather than high-fat alternatives.

Exercise

Don't forget the healing power of exercise during times of stress. It can lift your mood because it makes your body produce endorphins. It can help you lose weight by speeding up your metabolism and distracting you from food. It can help manage your stress hormones and give you feelings of pleasure and control.

Hopefully after reading this chapter you'll have the tools you need to zap bad habits that can stop you following your plan. Living with PCOS is a challenge and requires effort, but it can also be incredibly rewarding. Whether or not you're taking medication for PCOS, the diet and lifestyle recommendations in the Protection Plan can help you take charge of your health and improve your physical, mental and emotional well-being, now and in the years to come.

REFERENCES

1. Jahanfar, S. *et al.*, 'Bulimia nervosa and polycystic ovary syndrome', *Gynecol Endocrinol* 1995 Jun; 9 (2): 113–17
2. Michelmore, K. F. *et al.*, 'Polycystic ovaries and eating disorders: Are they related?', *Hum Reprod* 2001 Apr; 16 (4): 765–9
3. Seidenfeld, M. F. *et al.*, 'Impact of anorexia, bulimia and obesity on the gynecologic health of adolescents', *Am Fam Physician* 2001 Aug 1; 64 (3): 445–50
4. Coffey, S. *et al.*, 'The effect of polycystic ovary syndrome on health-related quality of life', *Gynecol Endocrinol* 2003 Oct; 17 (5): 379–86

14 In Partnership with the Professionals

66 *Luckily I had a doctor who warned me about the complications associated with PCOS and suggested I set up a plan of regular screenings to minimize my risk. But I know that not all doctors are that informed about PCOS, and it worries me that many women with PCOS simply aren't getting the information, support, screenings and advice they need.* 99

Carolyn, 30

Symptoms of PCOS should never be dismissed or ignored. 'PCOS carries with it potentially severe health risks,' says Dr James Douglas, PCOS expert and reproductive endocrinologist at the Plano Medical Center in Texas, 'and if you notice anything unusual about your appearance or have persistent menstrual cycle irregularity, it's in your best interests to see a doctor right away. Just because your symptoms are mild, this does not mean they should be ignored. You need to find out if you've got PCOS.'

So much more is known today about PCOS, and this gives us a big advantage as far as our long-term health is concerned. Keeping in close contact with your doctor offers an unparalleled opportunity to catch and prevent problems before they become serious. Regular check-ups and screenings can help you ward off PCOS-related diabetes, insulin resistance, cancer, heart disease and osteoporosis. Screening can also help determine whether or not you need medication as well as your healthy diet and lifestyle changes to minimize your long-term risks.

In this chapter we've put together a list of the most relevant screenings for women with PCOS. Ideally you should be screened every six months or at least once a year, more if you're overweight and insulin resistant. 'Screening for women with PCOS should be regular and appropriate for the individual.' says Dr Adam Balen, Professor of Reproductive Medicine and Surgery at Leeds General Infirmary.

BLOOD GLUCOSE/INSULIN LEVELS

'The data for the link between PCOS and diabetes is quite clear,' says PCOS expert Helen Mason, 'so informing the patient of this and regular screening really is a requirement.' Since PCOS is associated with an increased risk of developing insulin resistance and diabetes along, you and your doctor should keep a close eye on your blood sugar levels. Every year or so, ask your doctor for a glucose tolerance test (see page 16). There are home tests for glucose levels in the urine, but 'The only recommended method to diagnose diabetes accurately is by a blood test carried out by a doctor' says Natasha Eve from Diabetes UK.

BLOOD FAT ANALYSIS

Since high cholesterol is associated with PCOS, you need to have regular tests to measure your level – every six months if you are overweight; yearly if your weight is within the normal range. A high level of unhealthy cholesterol or an abnormal lipid profile contributes to the development of heart disease, especially if other risk factors are present. An LDL or 'bad' cholesterol level below 130 mg/dl is desirable. LDL levels of 130–159 mg/dl are borderline high. Levels of 160 mg/dl are high.

Cholesterol levels are checked through a simple blood test. You can also ask your pharmacist about the availability of home cholesterol tests – although do bear in mind that opinion is divided among doctors and pharmacists as to how useful and accurate these can be. 'Some tests cannot be relied on to make an accurate medical diagnosis,' says Dr

Catti Moss of the Royal College of General Practitioners. Generally, though, most doctors feel these tests can help as an early indicator – but if anything unusual shows up you need to see your doctor. 'Ideally cholesterol should be measured by the doctor or a practice nurse,' says Belinda Linden of the British Heart Foundation

BLOOD PRESSURE

With the increased risk of high blood pressure associated with PCOS you need to check yours every six months. This is relatively easy to do at home; there are many over-the-counter tests available. These home tests can and do provide a good general guide, but aren't always 100 per cent reliable so it's still important to get tested regularly by your doctor. 'We only recommend the use of upper arm digital monitors,' says Natasha Shepherd from the National Blood Pressure Association in the UK. For more information on blood pressure, what's healthy and what's not, refer back to page 39.

WEIGHT AND BODY FAT

With the increased risk of obesity and its related health problems associated with PCOS, you should keep a close eye on your weight. Similarly, being very underweight is not healthy and may have serious implications for developing conditions such as osteoporosis later in life.

Weighing yourself every week or so isn't always the best indicator of health. A more reliable indicator is your waist and hip measurements, as we know that a woman who is apple-shaped is at a greater health risk than a pear-shaped woman.[1] Measuring yourself around the hips and waist on a monthly basis if you're on a weight-loss programme, or every couple of months if you're not, can be very useful. For more information on body fat, the health risks associated with apples and pears and how to measure yourself correctly, see page 47.

Breast awareness

Get to know how your breasts feel and look so you can be alert to any changes. Doctors are more likely to detect problems, but being breast aware and regularly examining yourself is a plus. Do bear in mind that before and during your period your breasts may feel lumpier than usual, so the best time to check is typically in the week or so after your period has finished. A good way to check for any changes is to stand before a mirror and look at your breasts, bearing in mind that it is usual for one to be slightly bigger than the other. Check for any shape or skin changes or changes in your nipples. Raise your arms and turn from side to side. The more familiar you are with your breasts and the way they look from the front and side, the more likely you are to detect anything unusual.

Then, either still standing or lying down (which some women find easier), using a wet, soapy hand, make small circles with the flat of your middle three fingers from your armpit in towards the breast and your nipple to feel for unusual lumps or changes. Look for something that feels different from the usual bumpy texture, something the size of a small marble. Keep your movements light and don't press too hard.

BONE HEALTH

If you're at high risk (have an eating disorder or exercise intensively or have PCOS) you may want to ask your doctor for a bone scan for osteoporosis every two or three years.

CANCER

With the increased risk of endometrial and breast cancer associated with PCOS you should have a pap smear test every year or two to pick up possible cancerous changes in the cells lining the womb. If they're picked up early these abnormal cells can easily be removed by laser before they become dangerous. In addition to having your breasts examined once a year by a doctor or nurse you should also get into the habit of regular self-examination to check for any unusual lumps, bumps or changes. If you examine yourself and there's anything about your breast tissue, shape, or feel that you're worried about, consult your doctor.

PCOS MEDICATION: HOW IT CAN HELP CUT YOUR RISKS

There are lots of medications that can help treat your PCOS symptoms and help prevent long-term complications. It would take another book to list them all, so we're giving you just the main options here. Try not to let the number of medications daunt you – it actually means that there's a lot of help out there and if one type of drug isn't working for you, the chances are your doctor can help you find an alternative.

The key is getting a tailor-made prescription that works for you.

For example, acne might be your most troublesome problem, or it could be fertility problems, weight control, or insulin resistance – so each of these concerns would be treated with different medication.

So, once you have a PCOS diagnosis, you'll talk to your doctor about what will best work for you. They'll want to know if you're trying for a baby, as some medications aren't suitable if you are. But here are some of the most commonly used treatments you might be offered as part of your PCOS treatment plan.

Irregular periods

As we've discussed, the irregular periods associated with PCOS are linked to an increased risk of endometrial cancer. The normal, cyclic shedding of your womb lining (endometrium) which is controlled by the rise and fall of progesterone following ovulation doesn't work as normal if you don't ovulate, and so your womb lining can become abnormally thickened. Treating irregular periods is more than a matter of convenience as research shows that inducing regular bleeds in women with PCOS will lower the risk of developing endometrial cancer.[2]

Unless you're trying to get pregnant, the most common medication to induce regular periods is the birth-control pill. There are a large number of pills to choose from, each with a different blend of synthetic oestrogens and progestins (progestin is a synthetic form of progesterone).

The Pill is a reliable form of contraception that can reduce the risk of endometrial cancer, but you should be aware of the risks associated with the Pill if you've got PCOS. The British Medical Association's *Official Guide to Medicine and Drugs* lists blood sugar problems as a possible side-effect,[3] synthetic oestrogens can cause water retention (oedema) and increase the drive towards insulin resistance, progestins can increase appetite and may contribute to weight gain, not forgetting the much-publicized risk of blood clots, as well as high blood pressure, high cholesterol and perhaps even breast cancer. All these risk factors increase significantly if you're overweight and you smoke.

PCOS specialist Dr Adam Carey admits that when he worked in hospitals, he would routinely put women with the symptoms of PCOS on the Pill, though he now thinks that this approach not only fails to tackle the underlying condition but will actually make it worse in the long term. 'The symptoms will improve over the short term, say two to three years, but when they return they're likely to be even more severe because of the impact the contraceptive pill has on insulin production.'

Insulin, as you know, works to control sugar levels in the blood, and many women with PCOS are known to be resistant to their own insulin. 'It's as if the cells have gone deaf and can no longer pick up messages from the pancreas, which makes insulin, about how much is needed,' says Dr Carey. 'When this system breaks down, the body reacts by storing more of the calories from your food, especially carbohydrates, as fat. You put on weight, even though you're eating the same amount. Excess insulin also acts on the ovaries to make more testosterone – which is the very last thing you need. It's also the reason the contraceptive pill, which makes the body even more insulin resistant, is an ill-advised short-term solution.'

So if you've PCOS and are overweight but still feel the Pill is the best option for you, it's crucial that you follow a healthy eating, no-smoking, healthy living plan and communicate regularly with your doctor. And, however much your symptoms improve when you're on the Pill, bear in mind that the Pill only masks the symptoms of PCOS. Once you stop taking it, they are likely to return.

The permanent solution is to make healthy diet and lifestyle changes, with or without medication or the Pill – and of course to lose weight if you've got weight to lose.

If, however, you're aware of the risks and still want to take or stay on the Pill, you need to know which brands may affect PCOS and your long-term health the most.

Oral contraceptives come in two types: progesterone-only pills and the combined oral contraceptive pill containing oestrogen and proges-terone.

You would think that progesterone-only pills, which must be taken at the same time each day, would be the best choice as they will elimi-nate the chance of oestrogen-related side-effects and the drive towards insulin resistance. Yet it seems that many women find that progesterone-only pills don't properly suppress PCOS symptoms and can even make them worse. One study suggests that the progesterone-only pill produces the greatest risk of diabetes, which women with PCOS already have a risk of developing – along with oestrogen-progestin combinations containing strong progestins.[4] Of the contraceptives studied, the combination pill containing a substance called norethin-drome appeared to be the safest and did not increase the risk of diabetes. Do ask your doctor about this.

It seems that progestin-only pills can increase the androgenic (male hormone) effects of progesterone, which makes symptoms worse, so it makes sense to use oestrogen-progestin combinations that have the least androgenic activity. This narrows the field to choices such as Apri, Kariva, Desogen, Mircette, Ortho-Cept, Ortho-Cyclen, Ortho Tri-Cyclen and Ortho Tri-Cyclen Lo. These are the type most commonly prescribed for women with PCOS in the US. In the UK, Dianette is the least androgenic, and is often prescribed for unwanted facial and body hair — but it's worth mentioning that Dianette has been associated with the risk of blood clots and strokes. It's generally recommended that women switch to a lower-dose preparation such as Cilest or Yasmin, after six months — that is, once the symptoms of PCOS have been brought under control. You also shouldn't take Dianette if you've got diabetes or high blood pressure. 'If symptoms are severe and you're taking Dianette it's fine if it's monitored properly,' says Dr Balen, 'although the current advice is to switch to a lower-dose pill once symptoms are controlled.'

If you're prone to acne you need to go for contraceptive pills with the new progestins that are active on skin receptors (and also reduce the risk of weight gain) such as Minulet, Femodene, Ovysmen and Brevinor.

Some women feel better on the Pill than others. Each case is highly individual. It's a matter of looking at the benefits and risks and deciding with your doctor what best suits your individual needs. If you think the Pill is making your symptoms worse, tell your doctor immediately and switch to another brand. You may also find that if you've been taking one brand of Pill for several years your symptoms seem to be returning, perhaps as a result of increased insulin resistance. The best advice if you're taking the Pill is to proceed with caution and monitor things carefully, and of course to eat a healthy diet and to exercise regularly. Studies suggest that the Pill can leach valuable nutrients as well as alter mineral and vitamin levels,[5] so it's a good idea to supplement with extra zinc, B vitamins and folic acid to help your liver break down synthetic hormones effectively. You also need to check that your daily multivitamin and -mineral contains enough vitamin C and vitamin E.

If you don't want to take the Pill, another option for irregular periods is to induce cyclic shedding of the endometrium by prescribing progesterone on a regular basis. Professor Stephen Franks, PCOS expert and Professor of Reproductive Endocrinology at Imperial College, London, believes 'this is a very sensible alternative to taking a combined oral contraceptive pill to ease symptoms and regulate your cycle.' Just bear in mind that cyclic use of progesterone doesn't prevent ovulation, so it won't work as a contraceptive. Nor should you use it if you're trying for a baby.

For some women, however, the side-effects of progestin-only preparations can sometimes include weight gain, fluid retention and digestive problems. You'll need to see how you feel and whether it suits you or not.

Another option is a progesterone-releasing coil called Mirena. This type of coil can effectively prevent the abnormal build-up of the endometrium. It can cause light spotting, and occasionally periods can stop altogether, but because this occurs when the endometrium is thin it's considered safe. 'The Mirena coil is ideal for women with PCOS,' says Dr Balen. 'It releases progesterone into the womb and prevents abnormal thickening of the womb lining secondary to unopposed oestrogen production – which occurs in women with PCOS who are not ovulating. The Mirena should be changed every five years.'

Fertility problems

Infertility in women with PCOS is often due to lack of ovulation and infrequent or irregular periods. If this is the case, diet and lifestyle changes to help establish a normal cycle are typically recommended along with fertility drugs to prepare the ovaries for a better response to ovulation-inducing treatments and/or ovulation-inducing agents such as clomiphene. The use of insulin-sensitizers such as metformin have also be shown to improve outcomes. If these methods don't work, surgical techniques such as ovarian wedge resection or laparoscopic ovarian drilling may achieve the desired results.

The treatment of infertility in women with PCOS is complex and many-faceted, and outside the scope of this book. We've covered it in detail in *PCOS and Your Fertility*; the main thing we want to say here is, don't lose hope! There is a lot of help available to you, and there's so much you can do for yourself with a healthy diet and exercise programme. Around 70 per cent of women with PCOS do conceive naturally in the end, and for anyone taking fertility treatment the success rate is thought to be as high as 90 per cent.[6]

Unwanted facial and body hair and acne

Unwanted facial and body hair (hirsutism), hair loss (alopecia) and acne are the result of levels of testosterone that are too high. Testosterone levels are managed by the amount of SHBG in the blood. High levels of insulin lower the production of SHGB and so increase the levels of active testosterone.

Contraceptive pills such as Dianette or Yasmin are often prescribed for acne or hirsutism, but if these aren't effective a medication called Androcur, which contains cyproterone acetate, may be given alongside. The effect on acne is usually seen within a couple of months, but the effect on hirsutism and hair loss may take up to 18 months owing to the slow rate of hair growth. During that time you can use depilatory creams, electrolysis, laser treatments, waxing and shaving. As cyproterone can have a negative effect on your liver, liver function should be regularly checked, and you can help to boost its health yourself with the recommendations on page 106.

Spironolactone is another medication used to treat stubborn acne and hirsutism, but as the drug can cause irregular periods it's often given alongside the contraceptive pill. Spironolactone can reduce water tension and lower blood pressure in those with high blood pressure, and is often given when it's unsafe to give the Pill, for example in cases of obesity, high blood pressure or those who smoke.

Other anti-androgen medications aimed at hirsutism and taken alongside the contraceptive pill include flutamide and finasteride. Side-effects can include mood swings, loss of libido, fatigue and impaired liver function – so you need to make sure you and your doctor are monitoring your health while you take it.

Examples of anti-acne medications include topical cleansers, keratolytics such as benzoyl peroxide or azelaic acid to clear out pores, astringents to tighten pores, oral antibiotics to decrease skin bacteria and oral agents such as Retin A that alter the shedding of skin cells. An option for male-pattern hair loss is the use of topical Rogaine to stimulate hair growth. Although helpful, these interventions don't get to the core of the problem: excessive male hormones. The best way to correct the hormonal imbalance is, as we've stressed throughout this book, to take appropriate dietary measures, exercise regularly and lose weight if you've got weight to lose.

Obesity

If diet and exercise alone don't work, prescription weight-loss medications could help you. There are medications that can inhibit your body's absorption of fat from your diet, but since they inhibit good fats as well as bad they should only be used in the short term to start the progress of weight loss, or when all else has failed.

For more information on slimming drugs, see page 136.

Insulin resistance

The first line of attack as far as insulin resistance is concerned is weight loss. The next step is to consider taking a drug called metformin (glucophage) – an anti-diabetes drug that's used to treat Type II diabetes. Since insulin resistance is thought to be one of the underlying causes of PCOS, prescribing metformin can have dramatic and far-reaching effects. The use of metformin in women with PCOS has been shown to decrease androgen levels,[7] improve acne and hirsutism, normalize irregular periods, restore fertility, facilitate weight loss and prevent the progression to diabetes.

It seems as if the appropriate use of anti-diabetes insulin-lowering mediations such as metformin not only treats all the symptoms of PCOS, but also prevents many of the serious complications. Side-effects when taking metformin can include upset stomach, skin rashes, agitation, diarrhoea and flatulence, but these tend to subside in a few weeks unless you are increasing your dosage. Although no detrimental effects on pregnancy have been reported, you and your doctor may decide it's best to stop if you do get pregnant.

Although anti-diabetes medications have not yet been approved for use in the US or UK for PCOS patients, a few studies conducted into the use of insulin-lowering drugs as a treatment for PCOS suggest they may be beneficial for long-term health. They appear to regulate ovulation and sometimes there's an improvement in weight loss and blood cholesterol levels. But they're not a miracle cure for women with PCOS, says Professor Stephen Franks. 'There have been too few large-scale, properly conducted studies of the effects of metformin in PCOS to be able to make thorough conclusions.'

NATURAL THERAPIES

❝*I wasn't against medical treatment, I just wasn't sure I wanted to commit to a medication that I might have to take for the rest of my life. I didn't want to be a guinea pig for new drugs either, and preferred the natural approach. My doctor admitted he wasn't sure about natural treatments but was willing to help and support me as long as I got my insulin levels monitored regularly and had at least four periods a year. With my doctor's requirements in mind I visited a nutritionist, medical herbalist and reflexologist, and firmly believe that natural therapies have helped keep my symptoms under control and my periods regular for the last three years.*❞
Rebecca, 30

As well as improving your diet and lifestyle and starting a regular exercise routine, there is a whole range of natural therapies you can use to improve the quality of your life and your long-term health. These are usually free of side-effects and can be used alongside medication, in consultation with your doctor.

To help you begin your exploration, this section will explore some of the options that women have used to reduce the symptoms and stresses of PCOS and prevent the long-term risks associated with it.

Remember to inform your doctor if you're trying an alternative approach, and ideally get your nutritionist/natural therapist and your doctor to communicate with each other so you can make sure you're getting the best of both worlds and that each practitioner knows the full story – this can ensure that neither medication has a detrimental effect on the other, and also help more doctors and natural health practitioners find out about what works best for PCOS.

Herbal remedies

Many conventional modern medicines are made from plant-derived substances, and because herbal medicines tend to have few side-effects they are perhaps the most popular complementary therapy and preventative medicine for women with PCOS.

Although they're natural, however, you should still use herbal remedies with caution because they're very powerful. Always make sure you take advice from a trained herbalist and consult with your doctor to make sure they're not going to interfere with any prescribed drugs you're taking.

Let's take a look at some common herbal remedies used by women with PCOS.[8]

Agnus castus

This is a popular herbal medicine for women with PCOS and it has a long history of use for female hormone regulation. It appears to work with the pituitary gland, which stimulates the reproductive hormones into action. Research has shown that over a six- to eight-month period, Agnus castus can help normalize the menstrual cycle, balancing progesterone and oestrogen production and reducing the health risks associated with excess oestrogen, such as obesity and breast cancer.[9] Extracts from Agnus castus berries help to neutralize the excess testosterone occurring in PCOS, and may help to reduce acne and excess hair. It also decreases secretion of follicle-stimulating hormone (FSH) and increases production of luteinizing-hormone (LH). Because LH stimulates ovarian secretion of progesterone, Agnus castus helps to regulate the menstrual cycle, tending to shorten a long cycle and lengthen a short one. It's slow acting and takes an average of 25 days for symptoms to start improving, and as long as six months to achieve the full effect. Agnus castus can also increase fertility where difficulty in conceiving is linked with low progesterone levels during the second half of the menstrual cycle – but treatment should be stopped as soon as pregnancy is suspected, as it's not recommended during pregnancy and shouldn't be taken at the same time as other hormone treatments such as HRT or the Pill.[10]

Ashwaganda
Sometimes called Indian ginseng, ashwaganda is an adaptogenic herb. If you're under stress it can help your body to adapt. Although no research has been done for women with PCOS, studies show that it can boost sexual function,[11] raise energy levels, stabilize mood swings, decrease anxiety, aid the detoxification of hormones and increase your resistance to disease.

Astragalus
This is a tonic herb, frequently used in Traditional Chinese Medicine which is thought to aid adrenal function and boost your immunity and general health. It's also thought to improve nutrient absorption and speed up metabolism, thereby reducing the risk of obesity.

Bitter melon
Bitter melon is a herb that may help to normalize elevated blood sugar levels. It also holds great promise as a treatment for cancer.[12] Other Ayurvedic herbs believed to reduce the risk of diabetes include tulsi and Gymnema sylvestre.[13]

Black cohosh
Also known as Black Cohesh, this was widely used by Native Americans and colonial Americans for the relief of menstrual cramps and

menopausal symptoms. Studies show that the herb has substances that bind with oestrogen receptors and can help balance hormones.[14] An added benefit is that Black Cohosh can also slightly lower blood pressure and cholesterol levels, possibly reducing the risk of heart disease.

Cinnamon

Cinnamon, widely used in cooking, has been shown by research to help make fat cells more responsive to insulin, helping them to metabolize glucose.[15] A dash of cinnamon or half a teaspoon with every meal or appropriate dish may help keep blood sugar levels in check and diabetes and insulin resistance at bay.

Note: Don't use a lot of cinnamon if you're pregnant.

Dong quai

This is a Chinese herb, also called angelica, which is well known as a tonic for the female reproductive system, regulating hormones and improving menstrual regularity.[16]

Fenugreek

Together with Gymnema sylvestre, Fenugreek is a herb that seems to interfere with sugar absorption and improve insulin sensitivity, thereby helping to reduce the risk of diabetes. Fenugreek shouldn't be taken during pregnancy. According to Dr Ann Walker, medical herbalist and Senior Lecturer in Human Nutrition at the University of Reading, herbs can be a powerful force in balancing and reducing insulin levels in women with PCOS. When treating women with PCOS and insulin problems, as well as patients with diabetes, Dr Walker often uses fenugreek and Gymnema sylvestre as well as cinnamon, bilberry, and goat's rue.

Ginkgo biloba

This has been shown to increase blood flow to the brain, which can encourage clear thinking.[17] There isn't agreement on this, but some experts think that anyone with a circulatory problem – or at risk of developing one, as women with PCOS are – should take Ginkgo biloba.

St John's Wort
St John's Wort has been studied extensively and shown to help people with mild to moderate depression, as it can increase the action of the chemical serotonin without the side-effects associated with mood-boosting drugs such as Prozac.[18] It's also thought that St John's Wort can encourage sleep and boost the immune system. Its anti-inflammatory and antiviral properties can be useful for treating acne.

In addition to St John's Wort, other herbal remedies that can ease emotional stress – and stress, you may recall, is linked to an increased risk of poor health – include white peony, motherwort, chamomile, lavender, lemon balm and vervain. White peony is particularly useful for women with PCOS since, as well as helping to reduce stress and irritability, it can also help normalize androgen levels in the body.

Sairei-to
This Chinese herbal medicine may be a useful treatment for women with PCOS and irregular periods according to research at the Department of Obstetrics and Gynaecology at Nippon Kokan Hospital in Kagawa, Japan.[19]

Saw palmetto
This has been shown to be effective for male prostate problems, and it is thought that it may help counteract the effects of excess testosterone in women, such as acne and excess hair.

Siberian ginseng
Siberian ginseng is another adaptogenic herb that can improve hormone activity and sexual function, boost energy and physical performance under stress, reduce blood sugar fluctuations and increase resistance to disease.[20] It's frequently recommended to women with PCOS and has few side-effects.

Unkei-to

The Japanese herbal mixture Unkei-to is a blend of 12 herbs including ginseng,[21] evoida fruit and ginger stem that can help encourage ovulation in women with PCOS and improve menstrual regularity, thus reducing the risk of endometrial cancer.

Spagyric herbal remedies

Developed for women with PCOS who are hoping to conceive and cannot use saw palmetto to help redress their underlying hormone

---

Herbs for the heart

The following herbs are thought to lower blood pressure and reduce the risk of heart disease:[23]

- hawthorn tincture
- motherwort tincture
- dandelion root tincture
- raw garlic.

Just half a clove of raw garlic a day can dramatically reduce your blood pressure.[24] Garlic may also have a mild blood sugar-lowering effect and is linked with heart health because it contains a substance which can stimulate your body to produce HDL – the good cholesterol.

Blood thinners, such as aspirin, can reduce the incidence of stroke or heart attack. A daily spoonful of vinegar made from the leaves, buds and flowers of any of the following can give you the same health protection as aspirin, help calcium absorption and improve digestion, too:

- alfalfa
- birch
- sweet clover
- bedstraw
- red clover
- willow
- wintergreen.

Do not take blood-thinning herbs if you have heavy periods or will be having surgery in the near future.

imbalances, spagyric formulations ('spagyric' refers to when healing forces from nature, such as plants and minerals, are applied as remedies and display therapeutic effectiveness) include the root of an African plant called *Okoubaka aubrevillei*. This helps clear toxins, including hormonal metabolites, from the body, and can reduce the unexplained weight gain that is a common symptom of this hormonal disorder. It also includes *Sambucus nigra* (elder), which works specifically to correct hereditary disorders and in this instance reduce cysts. The most important ingredient, however, is *Dioscorea villosa*, or wild yam,[22] which acts as a hormone regulator to help restore a normal menstrual cycle and fertility.

The herbs listed above have been used with varying degrees of success by women with PCOS. It's very important to note, however, that the herbs have not been regulated by the US or UK governments for use on women with PCOS, so only consider using herbal remedies with your doctor's consent and the help of a trained professional.

Homoeopathic treatments

Because PCOS is so complex and symptoms differ from woman to woman, each woman will require a remedy or constitutional treatment that has been selected to treat her individually. This does not just include your period-related symptoms (in fact, these are often given the least emphasis), but all of the general facts about you: your personality, likes and dislikes, what foods you prefer or dislike, your sleep patterns, normal body temperature (this can vary slightly from woman to woman) and the weather/season, to name but a few. Once selected, the appropriate remedy is prescribed in a very short dosage regimen; this acts like a short, sharp shock to the body's energy system in order to get it vibrating at the right frequency which equates to health. Follow-ups to assess the result of the treatment are usually carried out four to five weeks later.

Constitutional (overall) remedies often prescribed for PCOS cases include Pulsatilla, Lycopodium, Sepia and Lachesis. Where there's evidence of hormonal imbalances that have not been corrected by the constitutional remedy, glandular remedies to stimulate the relevant endocrine glands may be used. Looking at the diet and nutritional state of the patient is also very important, and a homoeopath may refer you to a clinical nutritionist for a full assessment.

Aromatherapy

Aromatherapy uses the sense of smell in the treatment of certain health disorders alongside delivering the healing chemicals from plant oils into your bloodstream via your skin with massage (the oils are then absorbed in the same way as medication is absorbed through, say, a nicotine or HRT patch), or via diffusion through the air and the blood vessels in the lining of your nose. The aim of aromatherapy for PCOS is to normalize hormone imbalances and aid relaxation and the release of emotional stress.

Any therapy that lowers stress levels is a plus for women with PCOS, because the way the body responds when the mind perceives stress is to pump more cortisol and adrenaline out, which in turn raises glucose levels and worsens insulin resistance.

The oils thought to be particularly useful for women with PCOS are rose oil (which may help regulate menstrual cycles and boost confidence), geranium oil (which can help relieve anxiety) and clary sage (which can ease period problems and depression). Other helpful and calming oils include bergamot, jasmine, chamomile, lavender and neroli.

Aromatherapist Katherine Ginsberg, co-founder of The Birth Connection (www.birthconnection.co.uk), a group of London-based complementary therapists specializing in menstrual and fertility problems, explains that 'Essential oils are often balancing in their effects, helping the body to return from a state of imbalance which has led to illness to one of balance and health. This is one of the reasons why aromatherapy lends itself so well to the treatment of PCOS – which is all about the under- or over-production of various hormones. The work I do with my clients is often about bringing the body and mind back into balance. Once this has been achieved, the symptoms of PCOS will often improve. Moreover, when essential oils are breathed in they go directly to the brain, the control centre of the hormonal system.'

Acupuncture

Acupuncture has been used for thousands of years, and although an ancient therapy it is gaining more and more recognition from modern science for its ability to help with a range of health problems, for example headaches, stress, nausea and vomiting.[25] Although no specific studies have been done with PCOS as yet, many women we have talked to have found it helpful, especially with irregular periods and fertility problems. So how does it work?

Acupuncture involves stimulating the body's vital energy, or *chi*, at specific points located along energy channels called *meridians*. These meridians are believed to correspond to specific internal organs. Incredibly fine needles are inserted to unblock or increase the flow of *chi* so that the balance of Yin (the female force) and Yang (the male force) is restored.

Emotional, physical and environmental factors are thought to disturb the flow of chi energy balance. Acupuncture has been used to alleviate stress, asthma and allergies. It's also thought to be capable of kick-starting periods and helping to regulate menstrual cycles in women with PCOS.

Women with PCOS will probably have needles placed at points in their arms, legs and abdomen, and the acupuncturist will probably work on the liver and spleen *chi* to treat abdominal bleeding. Some people experience a stinging sensation when the needles go in, but for most people it's a painless procedure.

Autogenic therapy

Autogenic therapy has been used with success to treat physical and emotional symptoms of stress and illnesses exacerbated by stress.[26] It draws on the insights of meditation and is particularly useful for mild anxiety states. The techniques have been found to lower blood pressure and improve emotional balance, both of which are particularly helpful for women with PCOS.

A typical session involves a series of exercises designed to focus your mind on feelings of heaviness and warmth in the limbs, a calm heartbeat, easy natural breathing, abdominal warmth and cooling of the forehead. You repeat the exercises three times a day after meals for about 10 minutes each time.

Reflexology

Another therapy that can aid the release of stress is reflexology – or foot massage. Experts in this type of manipulative therapy claim that all the organs of the body are reflected in the feet, in a similar way to acupuncturists believing there are specific places where the *chi* can be influenced, all of which can be exploited in the prevention and treatment of any disorder. 'This is especially important if you've got PCOS,' say reflexologists Mike Edwards and Ashi Le Hunte who run the Harley Street Complementary Health Centre in London, 'because reflexology treats the underlying cause and encourages your body to perform at the best level possible.'

Reflexology is a popular choice for women with PCOS, not just as a stress-buster but also because it's wonderfully relaxing and thought to be able to help regularize periods and improve circulation. 'Reflexology is one of the most effective ways of rebalancing the entire endocrine system,' says UK-based reflexologist Jacqui Garnier (Garnier70@aol.com) who has PCOS herself and uses reflexology to help other women. 'It is particularly successful when used in combination with a healthy diet and lifestyle. As a balancing treatment it has been shown to have success rates as high as 88 per cent in infertility, it can regulate cycles, encourage ovulation and reduce the stress so often associated with coping with the symptoms of PCOS.'

Traditional Chinese medicine

Chinese medicine addresses imbalances in the body with the aim of preventing disease in the future. It's this that makes it particularly helpful for women with PCOS. It can help re-establish the proper functioning of the body and hormones with methods that are gentler and subtler than those of orthodox medicine. It has a whole range of therapeutic techniques at its disposal, including herbs, acupuncture and dietary changes. 'Treatment with a Chinese practitioner,' says PCOS expert and acupuncturist Jo George, who runs the Life Medicine Acupuncture and Herb Clinic in London, 'can provide women with PCOS with enough strength to make the necessary changes to our lifestyle. All of us can benefit from simple adjustments, and for many this can mean increased vitality, greater well-being, better hormonal balance and feeling more contented with our lives.'

Traditional Chinese Medicine (TCM) reports fantastic results with hormonal disturbances, including PCOS. Practitioner Zita West, a former National Health Service midwife in the UK who specializes in holistic health for women, says she has helped many PCOS sufferers with TCM and a combination of acupuncture and rebalancing herbal and vitamin supplements.

Preventative medicine

With so many alternative therapies available it can sometimes be difficult to choose one that will help you. The bottom line is that in the same way as you may well have to try a few different prescription medications or different brands of the contraceptive pill before you find the one that really works for you, you'll need to do the same with natural therapies. The only way to find out is to experiment and see what works for you. A good place to start is to think about which one appeals to you most, or makes most logical sense to you. Then see if any of your friends, acquaintances or colleagues have seen a practitioner they would recommend, and start there.

Both of us have found that natural therapies have been a great addition to our approach to PCOS, in addition to healthy eating, exercise and trying to detox and reduce stress. Even if you simply find that an aromatherapy massage or herbal tea at the end of the day can help you unwind and feel less stressed, it's a bit of icing on your healthcare cake that can really contribute to preventing health problems in the future.

REFERENCES

1. Janssen, I., 'Weight circumference and not BMI explains obesity-related health risk', *Am J Clin Nutr* 2004 Mar; 79 (3): 379–84
2. Balen, A. *et al.*, 'Polycystic ovary syndrome and cancer', *Hum Reprod Update* 2001 Nov-Dec; 7 (6): 522–5
3. British Medical Association, *Official Guide to Medicines and Drugs* (Dorling Kindersley, 1998): 147
4. University of Southern California School of Medicine, 'Mini-pill increases risk of chronic diabetes in women with history of diabetes during pregnancy', Aug 1998 (www.sciencedaily.com/releases/1998/08)
5. Tyrer, L. B., 'Nutrition and the Pill', *J Reprod Med* 1984 July; 29 (7 Suppl): 547–50; Theuer, R. *et al.*, 'Effects of oral contraceptive agents on vitamin and mineral needs', *J Reprod Med* 1972; 8 (1): 13–19
6. Thatcher, S., *PCOS: The Hidden Epidemic* (Perspectives Press): 179–216
7. Hundel, R. S. *et al.*, 'Metformin: new understandings, new uses', *Drugs* 2003; 63 (18): 1879–94; Barbieri, R. L. *et al.*, 'Metformin for the treatment of the polycystic ovary syndrome', *Minerva Ginecol* 2004 Feb; 56 (1): 63–79
8. Tesch, B. J. *et al.*, 'Herbs commonly used by women: an evidence-based review', *Am J Obstet Gynecol* 2003 May; 188 (5 Suppl): S44–55
9. Cahill, D. J. *et al.*, 'Multiple follicular development associated with herbal medicine', *Hum Reprod* 1994; 9: 1469–70
10. Propping, D. *et al.*, 'Treatment of corpus luteum insufficiency', *Zeitschr* 1987; 63: 932–3
11. 'Withania somnifera – monograph', *Altern Med Rev* 2004 Jun; 9 (2): 211–14
12. Jia, W., 'Anti-diabetic herbal drugs officially approved in China', *Phytother Res* 2003 Dec; 17 (10): 1127–34
13. Shapiro, K. *et al.*, 'Natural products used for diabetes', *J Am Pharm Assoc (Wash)* 2002 Mar-Apr; 42 (2): 217–26

14. 'The use of black cohosh to treat symptoms of menopause', *Fertil Steril* 2004 Mar; 81 (Suppl 2): 27–34

15. Kham, A. *et al.*, 'Cinnamon improves glucose and lipids of people with type 2 diabetes', *Diabetes Care* 2003 Dec; 26 (12): 3215–18

16. Chang, H. S. *et al.*, 'Medicinal plants: conception/contraception', *Adv Contracept Deliv Syst* 1994; 10: 355–63

17. Dong, L. Y. *et al.*, 'Anti-aging action of the total lactones of ginkgo on aging mice', *Yao Xue Xue Bao* 2004 Mar; 39 (3): 176–9

18. Mennini, T. *et al.*, 'The antidepressant mechanism of Hypericum perforatum', *Life Sci* 2004 Jul 16; 75 (9): 1021–7

19. Sakai, A. *et al.*, 'Induction of ovulation by Sairei-to for PCOS patients', *Endocr J* 1999; 46: 217–20

20. Bucci, L. R. *et al.*, 'Selected herbals and human exercise performance', *Am J Clin Nutr* 2000 Aug; 72 (2 Suppl): 624S–36S

21. Ushiroyama, T. *et al.*, 'Effects of unkei-to, an herbal medicine, on endocrine function and ovulation in women with high basal levels of luteinizing hormone secretion', *J Reprod Med* 2001 May; 46 (5): 451–6

22. Russel, L. *et al.*, 'Phytoestrogens: a viable option?', *Am J Med Sci* 2002 Oct; 324 (4): 185–8

23. Fugh, B. A. *et al.*, 'Herbs and dietary supplements in the prevention and treatment of cardiovascular disease', *Prev Cardiol* 2000 Winter; 3 (1): 24–32

24. Zhang, X. H. *et al.*, 'A randomized trial of the effects of garlic oil upon coronary heart disease risk factors in trained male runners', *Blood Coagul Fibrinolysis* 2001 Jan; 12 (1): 67–74; Quidwai, W. *et al.*, 'Effect of dietary garlic (Allium sativum) on the blood pressure in humans – a pilot study', *J Pak Med Assoc* 2000 Jun; 50 (6): 204–7

25. Claraco, A. E. *et al.*, 'The reporting of clinical acupuncture research: what do clinicians need to know?', *J Altern Complement Med* 2003 Feb; 9 (1): 143–9

26. Ernst, E. *et al.*, 'Autogenic training for stress and anxiety: a systematic review', *Complement Ther Med* 2000 Jun; 8 (2): 106–10; Kanji, N. *et al.*, 'Management of pain through autogenic training', *Complement Ther Nurs Midwifery* 2000 Aug; 6 (3): 143–8

15 When Problems Arise

If your healthcare provider feels you're more at risk of one of the complications associated with PCOS than another due to family history, previous history as a smoker and so on, or your tests reveal that a related health problem has taken hold, then on top of your basic healthy protection plan lifestyle, and any current medication, there are a number of proven medications and supplements you and your doctor can consider. This chapter focuses on the problems that can emerge, and what you can do to help yourself.

HIGH CHOLESTEROL/ABNORMAL LIPID PROFILE

66 *I've got PCOS and abnormal cholesterol levels along with insulin resistance. It's scary stuff. My grandmother recently died of a heart attack. She'd had abnormal cholesterol for years, and ever since I can remember she was poorly. Thank goodness I have the chance to do something about it all and stop history repeating itself. My daughter's just had a little baby girl, and I want her to get to think of her Nana as someone who is healthy and vibrant.* 99

Moira, 44

Lipid is the collective name for biologic fats such as cholesterol, lipoproteins and triglycerides. High levels of triglycerides and high levels of low-density lipoproteins (LDLs, often referred to as 'bad' cholesterol) and/or low levels of high-density lipoproteins (HDLs, often referred to as 'good' cholesterol) are associated with an increased risk of heart disease in the future. (For more information about healthy cholesterol levels see pages 32–33.)

As we've seen, if you've got PCOS your risk of an abnormal lipid profile increases. Women with PCOS often have high LDL and triglyceride levels and low HDL levels, so much so that LDL levels can serve as a form of secondary diagnosis of the disorder. As there are no warning signs of high LDL cholesterol levels, every woman with PCOS should consider having a lipid profile performed at least once a year.

When symptoms appear, they usually take the form of angina or heart attack in response to the build-up of atherosclerotic plaque in the arteries. In the words of Dr Samuel Thatcher, PCOS expert and consumer advocate serving on the advisory board of the American Infertility Association, 'This is definitely a condition where it pays to invest in preventative medicine before dangerous complications occur.'

The best defence is, of course, diet and lifestyle changes as recommended in the Protection Plan. Stop smoking, reduce your intake of saturated fats, increase your intake of fibre, omega 3 and omega 6 essential fatty acids and exercise regularly. All these positive lifestyle changes can help protect against high levels of LDL and promote HDL formation. Some experts also advocate supplemental vitamin E and aspirin. Vitamin E is thought to help attack free radicals – harmful substances that promote LDL and reduce oxidative stress. Aspirin, taken in daily small doses, does not alter free radicals but it can help prevent clots from forming on damaged vessel walls.

An Aspirin a Day?

If you aren't at extremely high risk and don't have a documented history of heart disease, it probably isn't wise to take an aspirin a day as there's strong data to show that aspirin is poorly tolerated by a lot of women, with gastrointestinal bleeding being a major side-effect.

A cup or two of ginger tea a day may be a good alternative. Ginger makes blood less sticky and has some cholesterol-lowering ability.

Use of lipid-lowering drugs will usually only be recommended by your doctor if diet and lifestyle intervention, supplemental aspirin and vitamin E don't achieve target lipid levels in six months. Even if drugs are recommended, dietary therapy should continue to ensure maximum lipid lowering.

The kind of treatment your doctor suggests will depend on your LDL levels and the number of risk factors you have in addition to PCOS. In general, though, if LDL remains at 160 mg/dl or higher, drug therapy should be considered alongside your dietary and lifestyle changes.

There are a number of lipid-lowering drugs available which interfere with the processing of cholesterol. These are strong drugs, however, and ought to be a last resort. It's important to ask all about the potential side-effects, which can include gastrointestinal problems, allergic reactions, blood disorders and depression.

Prescription drugs for high cholesterol

Niacin (vitamin B₃)

In 1986 the Coronary Drug Project (a US National Institute of Health Study) found that prolonged use of niacin significantly reduced mortality rates among heart attack victims.[1] It has since become one of the most popular cholesterol-lowering drugs on the market. Because the dosage is up to 75 times higher than the recommended daily allowance, side-effects such as itching, flushing and panic attacks are common. Despite its popularity, niacin isn't a good choice if you've got PCOS, as it can increase insulin resistance.

Cholestyramine

This is considered the safest of the cholesterol-lowering drugs, but although it can lower LDL levels it can sometimes raise triglyceride levels, interact with other medication and trigger a host of unpleasant side-effects including really bad wind. Again, not the best choice if you've got PCOS.

Gemfibrozil

This drug lowers cholesterol and triglyceride levels in the blood, but there could be an increased risk of gallstone formation and muscle weakness. Commonly the taste of food is also altered, and bad wind may occur.

Statins

The cholesterol-lowering medication that stands out for women with PCOS is the 'statin' class of drugs. These have the potential to reduce the number of deaths from heart disease significantly without a whole host of undesirable side-effects. Statins have become the preferred treatment of abnormal lipid profiles for women with PCOS and insulin resistance.[2]

Statins, or HMG-CoA reductase inhibitors, can lower LDL cholesterol by inhibiting the enzyme that promotes cholesterol function. Pravastatin is the first statin to have US FDA approval for the role it plays in reducing the stickiness of the vessel walls and the likelihood of fat deposits on the vessel walls. It's likely that others will follow.

It's important to sound a note of caution, though, as – with the exception of pravastatin and fluvastatin – possible side-effects of statin use include muscle pain, tenderness and weakness. Studies also suggest that certain statin drugs, such as Lipitor, Zocor, Crestor and Pravachol, deplete stores of co-enzyme Q10. Low levels of co-enzyme Q10 have been associated with an increased risk of breast and cervical cancer. It's important that women with an increased risk of these cancers, as women with PCOS have, understand the association with statin drugs and ask their doctor about taking Co-Q10 supplements if they must be on a statin drug, to see if the benefits outweigh the risks and also to make sure they are monitored on a regular basis. Statins should also not be used if you're pregnant or trying for a baby.

Non-prescription supplements

If you're thinking of taking non-prescription drugs for high cholesterol, make sure you discuss this with your doctor and/or nutritionist or dietician first.

Arginine
Preliminary studies show that this amino acid may lower cholesterol levels and improve coronary blood flow by acting as an antioxidant and maintaining elasticity in blood vessel tissues.[3]

Turmeric
Turmeric assists hugely in the body's efficient management of cholesterol. It can be taken in capsules or as powder in drinks, and also cuts the risk of arteries hardening and high blood pressure.

Guggul
This Ayurvedic remedy contains substances called gugulipids which have been shown to have a major impact on the treatment of heart disease and diabetes. What makes gugulipids so important is that they're one of the very few compounds to regulate all fats in the body. As a result they can, over a three- to six-month period, help lower levels of bad cholesterol and raise levels of good cholesterol.

Co-enzyme Q10
Japanese and European practitioners love this powerful antioxidant, and a growing number of studies are offering support for its reputed ability to help the heart pump more efficiently and lower cholesterol.[4]

Alpha lipoic acid
A universal antioxidant that can improve blood sugar and insulin release, alpha lipoic acid may also help regenerate L-glutathione, an essential nutrient that helps deter atherosclerosis.

N-acetylcysteine (NAC)
NAC also helps to raise levels of L-glutathione. You may be wondering: why not take glutathione supplements instead? This is discouraged because glutathione is difficult to absorb.

Flavonoids

Studies have found that a higher intake of flavonoids reduces the risk of heart disease and atherosclerosis.[5] Red wine, green tea and grape seed and juice contain flavonoles, a subcategory of flavonoids that have been shown to help increase HDL, inhibit blood-clotting and prevent heart attack and stroke. You can find grapeseed extract and pinebark extract in your local health food store.

Other supplements that could prove helpful if you've an abnormal lipid/cholesterol profile include fenugreek (see page 104), chromium (see page 108) and vitamin E (see page 107).

HYPERTENSION

66 *On top of PCOS I've got hypertension. My doctor suggested that I make diet and lifestyle changes before trying medication. A friend of mine is on medication for hypertension, and although her blood pressure has improved she has noticed that she gets tired more often than usual and doesn't feel quite herself. I'm not sure if the tiredness is due to her frantic lifestyle or her blood pressure medication, but I'm definitely going to give the diet and exercise guidelines my doctor suggested a try before I take the drug option.* 99

Francesca, 38

The treatment and prevention of high blood pressure, or hypertension, also begins with the diet and lifestyle changes recommended in our Protection Plan: stop smoking, eat healthily, lose weight if you've got weight to lose, and exercise more.

Once again, medication isn't usually considered until at least a six-month trial of healthy diet and regular exercise has been attempted. It's especially important to make sure your diet is adequate in essential antioxidant substances such as vitamins C, E, A and B, zinc, selenium, etc., as these all help protect against free radical damage to the arteries, a major cause of high blood pressure.

If you need drug therapy there are a variety of antihypertensive drugs available; but unfortunately none of them is perfect. Most studies have been done on men and older women; more studies need to be done on women under the age of 50. You may find that you have to try several different drugs to find the one that best suits you.

Generally, once you start blood pressure medication you need to stay on it for the rest of your life, even after your blood pressure returns to normal. If you were to stop treatment, your reading would probably climb right back to an unhealthy level. The good news is that you may be able to reduce your dosage – once your blood pressure stays in the normal range (120/80) for at least a year.

Bearing this in mind, let's take a closer look at the most popular categories of blood pressure drugs your doctor may prescribe, and what side-effects they may cause.

Prescription drugs for high blood pressure
Diuretics
The drugs in this category lower blood pressure by flushing sodium and water from the body, which reduces the amount of sodium in your body. Generally doctors will prescribe diuretics in combination with other blood pressure medications.

Diuretics can deplete your body's potassium supply, causing fatigue, weakness and leg cramps. To compensate, drug companies have developed potassium-sparing diuretics such as spironolactone (Aldactone) and amiloride (Midamor). As their name suggests these drugs don't affect your body's potassium levels. The most common side-effects of potassium-sparing diuretics are stomach upset, diarrhoea, nausea and vomiting, mouth dryness and increased thirst. Spironolactone may be the best option for a diuretic if you have PCOS, as it's also an anti-androgen and used in the treatment of hirsutism.

Alpha-blockers (Cardura, Minpress)
These work by dilating blood vessels and decreasing resistance. The main side-effect can be a feeling of dizziness. They may be a good choice

for women with PCOS, although experts at the US National Heart, Lung and Blood Institute advise against using alpha-blockers as a first-line treatment in cases of high blood pressure with no complications.

Calcium channel-blockers

As their name implies these drugs (e.g. Norvasc, Plendil and Cardizem CD) prevent calcium from entering the muscle cells in your blood and heart vessels. This action allows the blood vessels to relax.

Side-effects include ankle swelling, constipation, headaches and a possible reduction in fertility.

Beta-blockers

These block the effects of adrenaline and widen blood vessels, slow the pulse and ease the heart's pumping action. Typically, beta-blockers are the first choice of therapy for uncomplicated hypertension. Older varieties such as propanolol had more side-effects than the newer, more selective beta-blockers such as Tenormin, Zebeta and Lopressor. One possible side-effect may be a lowering of libido and feelings of fatigue, but more significantly for women with PCOS beta-blockers can worsen glucose tolerance and lipid profiles. It's possible that they may not be the best choice if you've got PCOS.

Angiotensin converting enzyme (ACE) inhibitors

ACE inhibitors (e.g. Lotensin, Accupril, Monopril, Zestril and Captopril) reduce the production of angiotensin, a chemical that causes the arteries to constrict. The side-effects range from a dry throat and/or cough to skin rash. They are the drug of choice for women with insulin resistance/diabetes, and therefore probably the best choice if you've got PCOS.[6]

Non-prescription supplements for hypertension

Certain herbs and supplements may lower blood pressure as effectively as prescription pharmaceuticals, especially in combination with the lifestyle strategies we recommend in the Protection Plan. Even better, natural remedies tend to have fewer side-effects than drugs. On the other hand they do work more slowly than conventional medications, and can sometimes cause troublesome interactions with other drugs. For these reasons, always consult a doctor who is knowledgeable about herbs and nutritional supplements before adding them to your self-care regime.

Garlic

Studies have proven that garlic can help lower blood pressure.[7] For normal blood pressure, a clove of garlic every day can help keep it that way. If you've got high blood pressure, taking four to six 600 mg garlic capsules or tablets every day can help. If you don't like eating it you can always take a supplement – there are lots on the market now that have an anti-garlic breath coating, too!

Note: Because garlic thins the blood it should be used with caution if you're on prescription anti-coagulants or scheduled for surgery.

Co-enzyme Q10

This serves as a catalyst for the cellular reactions that support the production of ATP, the energy source for cells. ATP juices up the heart muscle cells, which pump with greater efficiency and less effort, which in turn helps lower blood pressure.[8] The recommended dosage is 100 mg a day taken with meals.

Onion

Not as effective as garlic but it can have similar benefits for lowering blood pressure. Cook with onions or take 2 or 3 tablespoons of onion oil a day.

Fish oil

Scientists aren't sure how fish oil lowers blood pressure and protects against heart disease, but it may have something to do with fish oil's ability to thin the blood, thus reducing the risk of clots.[9] You can get fish oil straight from the source, in fatty fish like salmon and tuna, or in fish oil supplements.

Chromium

If dietary chromium is low, then high blood pressure appears to develop more rapidly – probably because chromium is necessary for the use and production of insulin which controls levels of sugar in the blood. The precise link isn't clear, but the fact is that there's a demonstrable lack of chromium in individuals who die of heart disease. If you're hypertensive, 400–800 mcg chromium picolinate daily may be beneficial.

Calcium

You probably know about getting enough calcium to help protect against osteoporosis, but did you know it can also help rein in high blood pressure? A growing number of doctors are convinced that calcium has anti-hypertensive effects. Your best bet is to eat calcium-rich foods such as low-fat dairy products, fruits and vegetables, and to make sure your daily multivitamin and -mineral contains enough calcium.

Potassium

This can help by discouraging LDL cholesterol from sticking to artery walls. You can get a good amount of potassium just by eating a banana a day, but it's important to make sure, too, that your daily multivitamin and -mineral includes potassium.

Ginkgo biloba

It may be known as 'the brain herb', but ginkgo has cardiovascular benefits as well. It dilates the peripheral blood vessels – and any substance that does that can lower blood pressure by giving the blood more room to move. While ginkgo rarely causes side-effects it can inhibit the blood's ability to clot and is not recommended if you're taking a blood-thinning medication such as a daily aspirin.

Evening primrose oil

The oil from evening primrose contains gamma-linoleic acid, an essential acid that helps lower blood pressure. You can buy capsules containing the oil; follow the label instructions for proper use.

Hawthorn

Hawthorn is one of the most commonly recommended herbs for hypertension.[10] It's very potent and without the side-effects of conventional drugs. To treat high blood pressure, look for hawthorn capsules that are standardized as a flavonoid called vitexin, and follow the label's instructions for use. You can also buy hawthorn tincture, though this isn't as potent as the capsules.

Be sure to keep a close eye on your blood pressure, and limit your use to just a few weeks, unless you are taking it under medical supervision.

Other herbs and supplements that are commonly suggested and can have a beneficial effect on blood pressure include:

- dill seeds – contain an oil that acts as a diuretic (helping eliminate fluid from the body, reducing blood volume and lowering blood pressure)
- the herb devil's claw
- reishi (mushroom) capsules.

Finally, although not a supplement but a nutritious and calorie-free food, celery deserves a special mention as it may contain substances (3-n-butyl phthalide) that can help lower blood pressure. Add celery to salads, soups and meat or fish dishes, or use with vegetable dips.

INSULIN RESISTANCE/DIABETES

❝I *was diagnosed with diabetes on the day before my 39th birthday. Blood tests showed a fasting blood sugar level of 263, more than double the*

126 that's considered diabetic. The news wasn't a big surprise for me. After all, I had PCOS and had been insulin resistant for years, and both Type I and Type II diabetes run in my family. And I knew I was carrying more weight than I should, at 22 stone (308 lb) for my 5 foot 9 frame. My doctor suggested metformin along with a diet and exercise regime. Within a year I felt a whole lot better and had lost 11 stone (154 lb). I also met with a diabetes educator and nutritionist. The first thing she did was empty my fridge at home. After about five months I lost my taste for foods like rich meats and chocolate and found that I actually preferred lean meats and vegetables. I also launched into a walking programme — 30 minutes a day every day — and the pounds melted away. These days my blood sugar hovers in the near-normal range. I work hard to eat healthful foods and exercise regularly, because I want to protect my body from the complications PCOS and diabetes can cause. I've seen the complications in my family. One of my uncles ended up blind and the other died of a stroke. I'm not getting off scot free — I already have some kidney damage — but if I keep my blood sugar at a near-normal range I can reduce my chances of developing further complications. Metformin gives me the protection I need, but it's the diet and lifestyle changes that really make me feel better physically and emotionally. 99

Debbie, 40

The first treatment stage for insulin resistance/diabetes will always be to follow the diet and lifestyle recommendations as set out in the Protection Plan. The next step will be to consider a drug called metformin (glucophage) — an anti-diabetes drug that's often used to treat non-insulin-dependent or Type II diabetes.

For women with PCOS, metformin has been shown to lower levels of insulin and testosterone.[11] As a result, menstruation is often regulated and the symptoms of androgen excess (hirsutism, acne, etc.) may decrease.

Another good effect when metformin is combined with healthy diet and exercise is that it can help you lose weight (though it isn't guaranteed to have that effect on you).

'Although some women lose weight on metformin it's important to remember that metformin is not designed to help you lose weight,' says Dr Adam Balen, Professor of Reproductive Medicine and Surgery at Leeds General Infirmary. 'There are indications that it may improve metabolism and aid weight loss combined with appropriate diet and plenty of exercise, but the more overweight you are, the less likely metformin is to work.'

All in all, metformin does have benefits for both your long- and short-term health and is an effective treatment for insulin resistance/diabetes. It can also be combined with other medications such as blood pressure- and cholesterol-lowering drugs, but it isn't a cure. It's important to remember that diet and lifestyle changes are still essential. According to Gerard Conway, consultant gynaecologist at Middlesex Hospital, London, who has been working with women with PCOS to manage insulin resistance and improve symptoms using the drug metformin, 'Metformin is not a magic bullet and can only work if diet and exercise plans are already in place.'

Metformin treatment can be long term, but although often prescribed for women with PCOS who are insulin resistant, it isn't a licensed treatment for women with PCOS and can only be prescribed by an endocrinologist or specialist in reproductive medicine. Side-effects include upset stomach, flatulence, skin rashes and infections, but these usually subside after the first week or two.

Your doctor may also wish to prescribe other insulin-lowering drugs such as Actos (pioglitazone) or Avandia (rosiglitazone) either alongside metformin or in place of it. These medications have similar side-effects and, like metformin, can not only lower insulin but improve weight and blood cholesterol levels and help regulate periods.

If you're prescribed insulin-lowering medication, your doctor will want to discuss the options open to you, but whether you're prescribed metformin or another type of medication, be sure you know what it is you're being given and why.

Non-prescription treatments

You know we're going to say it, but we'll say it anyway — the crucial things for lowering insulin resistance are a healthy diet and exercise as part of the Protection Plan. Having said this, there are certain key nutritional supplements you could take to top up the effects of the Plan:

- Alpha lipoic acid. Studies on rats have shown that alpha lipoic acid can increase the efficiency of insulin.[12] Dosages ranging from 100 to 300 mg daily may be beneficial — although people with diabetes are likely to benefit from a higher dose — around 600 mg daily.
- Vitamin E can improve glucose control and manage insulin. To help reverse insulin resistance, take 400–800 IU daily.
- Chromium's key benefit is that it helps insulin function more efficiently.[13] If you've got insulin resistance or diabetes, 400–800 mcg of chromium picolinate daily can be helpful — but if you're on medication you need to monitor your glucose levels carefully to avoid over-medicating yourself.
- Zinc plays a crucial role in glucose regulation and the proper function of insulin. 30 mg daily is a good dose to start with.
- Magnesium is important for the normal function of insulin. Recommended dose: 400 mg daily.
- Manganese also plays a role in lowering blood glucose levels. Up to 30 mg daily may prove beneficial.

Polyphenols and flavonoids

These are plant-based compounds with powerful antioxidant properties and can play a big part in regulating blood sugar irregularities. They are found in citrus fruits and brightly coloured berries, green vegetables and (the best sources) green tea, bilberries, milk thistle extract, buckwheat, hawthorn berry and red wine.

Herbal supplements

Milk thistle

In the past few years there's been growing interest in silymarin (milk thistle) for regulating glucose levels, improving insulin resistance and other diabetes symptoms.[14] As with most herbs, the dosage must be tailored individually so you need to consult a trained medical herbalist for advice. Generally, if you're insulin resistant you'll need around 200 mg daily. If you have diabetes, you'll need 600 mg of silymarin daily.

Bitter melon

Bitter melon is technically a fruit, not a herb. It's commonly sold in Asian grocery stores and has impressive glucose-lowering effects as well as helping to reduce the symptoms of diabetes. Use the unripe, not the ripe fruit, to treat elevated glucose and diabetes. If you prefer supplements you can purchase these at any health food store.

Fenugreek

Fenugreek has a long history of use in Indian cooking and in Ayurvedic medicine for the treatment of diabetes and heart disease. Studies have shown that fenugreek seed powder can also lower glucose levels and improve a person's cholesterol profile.[15] The seeds are about 50 per cent fibre, which slows digestion and the post-meal rise in glucose levels. You can add fenugreek seed powder to food you prepare or drink it in a glass of water. If you prefer supplements, to improve glucose control 5–10 grams of fenugreek extract daily may prove beneficial.

Pycnogenol

New research from the Institute of Pharmaceutical Chemistry at the University of Muenster shows that Type II diabetes patients had lower blood sugar and healthier blood vessels after supplementing with French maritime pine tree bark extract, Pycnogenol. Between 50 and 200 mg of pine tree bark extract daily has been shown to not only lower glucose levels but to improve cardiovascular problems related to diabetes as well as reduce high blood pressure and cholesterol.

Gymnema sylvestre

This is another herb from India's Ayurvedic medical tradition that has been used for centuries to normalize excess sugar. Research has shown that it can increase the efficiency of insulin in reducing glucose levels.[16]

Gymnema is very bitter, so it's best to take supplements. To help glucose tolerance and insulin resistance, take 75–150 mg of standardized Gymnema extract daily.

Colosolic acid

This is an extract of the leaves of a Philippine plant. Research by Japanese scientists suggests that it's a promising herbal supplement for insulin resistance as it has an insulin-like effect and can lower glucose levels.[17]

Culinary herbs and spices

If you need yet another reminder to use less salt and pepper and to use herbs and spices instead, consider their glucose-lowering properties. Laboratory experiments by the US Department of Agriculture have found that garlic, cinnamon, cloves and bay leaves can improve insulin sensitivity, and that coriander can reduce glucose levels. Rather than search for these herbs in your health food store, simply add them to foods you bake. A pinch here and there contributes to your dietary protection against insulin resistance and diabetes, so eat as much as you – or those around you – can stand!

WEIGHT LOSS

❝Although metformin was prescribed for my PCOS I'm convinced that it's helped me to lose weight. Pre-metformin nothing I did seemed to shift the pounds, but as soon as I started metformin I lost six pounds. This was the boost I needed and, spurred on by the initial weight loss, I started to watch what I ate and exercise regularly. I've never felt so slim and fit.❞

Sue, 38

66 *Slimming pills may work for some women with PCOS but they were bad news for me. I lost my appetite completely. Yes, I did lose nearly 2 stone (25 lb), but as soon as I stopped taking them I got these huge cravings and not only did the weight pile back on again I gained even more weight than I had lost.* **99**

Mary, 33

Weight-loss drugs are now available that can inhibit the absorption of fat from the food you eat. However, many of these inhibit good fats as well as bad, and they should only be used when all else has failed and only in the short term to kick-start weight loss.

As far as weight management is concerned there's no substitute for a healthy diet and exercise weight-loss program, according to the guidelines we've given you earlier in this book.

Prescription weight-loss drugs

Slimming drugs that are based on amphetamines (speed) and thyroxine (animal hormones) either put you off food or increase your metabolic rate by increasing your heart rate. If you've got PCOS, you should avoid these completely.

Having said that, if your doctor feels that your weight carries with it a serious threat to your health unless you take a short-term diet drug, then it can be a useful stepping-stone – as long as you don't see it as a short-term measure in combination with a health diet. 'Slimming pills like Reductil,' says PCOS expert Adam Balen, 'can be useful sometimes if self-help measures have failed and they work the same way in PCOS as in any overweight woman.'

Slimming drugs should only ever be considered as a last resort when diet and lifestyle change hasn't worked. They are most effective when weight loss is combined with a healthy diet. The priority should always be to establish long-term healthy eating patterns. Although further studies need to be done on the effects of slimming drugs on women with PCOS, one slimming drug in particular could prove beneficial in the short term for obese women with PCOS. A study in Turkey suggests that the anti-obesity drug sibutramine (prescribed as Reductil) improves clinical and metabolic parameters in obese women with PCOS.[18] Hirsutism, excess weight, insulin sensitivity and BMI all improved after treatment with the drug.

Reductil works by tricking your brain into making your feel full and, unlike other drugs for obesity like Exenical (which prevents fat from being absorbed by the body), does not seem to have any side-effects. Research suggests an average weight loss of 20 lb over a six-month period.

Metformin isn't a slimming drug but an insulin-lowering drug often prescribed for insulin resistance and diabetes. Many women with PCOS who take metformin, however, notice that there's also an improvement in their weight.

Non-prescription treatments

For information on vitamins, minerals and nutritional supplements recommended to aid weight loss, see pages 106–9. There are also a number of herbal supplements you may want to take, but be sure to consult your doctor or a trained dietician and nutritionist first, as certain herbal supplements can be toxic in large doses.

Herbal supplements that could prove useful for women with PCOS who need to lose weight include:

- Fennel – a natural appetite suppressant
- Fenugreek – slows digestion and the post-meal rise in glucose
- Astragalus – increases energy and improves nutrient absorption
- Butcher's broom, cardamom, cayenne, cinnamon, garcinia carbogia, ginger, green tea and mustard seed – can improve digestion and aid in the metabolism of fat. (*Note:* Don't use cinnamon if you're pregnant.)
- Avoid any herbal slimming aids that contain ephedra, such as Metabolife 356, as research is suggesting it may have a potentially lethal effect on the heart. Ephedra is about to be banned in the US due to safety concerns.

SYNDROME X

❝*I'm overweight and got the lot — PCOS, hypertension, insulin resistance and wild blood sugar and cholesterol levels. My doctor saw my health problems as a disconnected group of symptoms and treated each separately. I was given a hypertensive drug for blood pressure, a stimulant to help me lose weight and a statin drug to help lower cholesterol. I never started to feel better and the drugs gave me unpleasant side-effects that left me feeling worse. As I turned the corner into my forties I saw my father, who had diabetes, die, my sister die of weight-complicated disease and my brother diagnosed with diabetes. I figured out that I was probably next. At 47 and still feeling unwell I read a newspaper article that described my condition as Syndrome X. Dietary changes were recommended. Though it was tough at first to break old habits, to my surprise after just two days I felt more energetic. After a week I had lost several pounds with very little effort. Surprised and encouraged, I've kept to my diet. My periods have returned — which was a shock as I thought I'd been through menopause. I really feel I've found the answer to my problems.* ❞

Janet, 47

Wouldn't it be easy if your doctor could write you a prescription for a drug to prevent or treat the cluster of symptoms that make up Syndrome X? This drug could improve how your body handles glucose, burn off extra weight, lower cholesterol and reduce your blood pressure. Unfortunately there isn't a magic pill that can do all that, so that many people with Syndrome X can end up taking several kinds of drugs, for example, beta-blockers for high blood pressure, statins to lower cholesterol, Reductil to lose weight, metformin to combat insulin resistance and so on. Trouble is, these drugs focus chiefly on the symptoms, not the underlying cause of Syndrome X, which is nutritional, and they may even increase your risk of other diseases. Given this situation the use of pharmaceutical drugs for Syndrome X is far from an ideal solution.

Since Syndrome X is a nutritional disease – caused primarily by the consumption of refined sugars and other carbohydrates – it makes sense to treat it with diet and lifestyle changes as we've recommended in the Protection Plan, instead of pharmaceutically. There are also a number of nutritional supplements which could prove helpful but, as with any kind of supplements that you take, they work best when integrated into a broad health program.

Alpha lipoic acid

This vitamin-like nutrient is found in many foods, including spinach, broccoli and beef. Of all the supplements, it could be the most important in helping to prevent and reverse Syndrome X. Its principal role is to help burn glucose, converting this sugar to energy that powers your heart, brain and every other organ. It also serves as one of the most distinctive antioxidant supplements, protecting the body against free radical damage. Research has shown that alpha lipoic acid can help normalize glucose and insulin levels in those with diabetes. The role it plays in converting glucose to energy is crucial to its role in correcting insulin resistance and Syndrome X.[19]

To help prevent Syndrome X, 50 mg of alpha lipoic acid daily may be beneficial. To reverse problems relating to glucose intolerance and Syndrome X, dosages ranging from 100 to 300 mg of alpha lipoic acid daily could prove helpful. Those with diabetes are likely to benefit from 600 mg daily, but they should only take this high dose under the guidance of their doctor.

Vitamin E

Like alpha lipoic acid, vitamin E influences glucose and insulin levels. However it plays a much more significant role as an antioxidant that counteracts many of the unwanted health effects of free radicals. By stemming the formation of free radicals, vitamin E reduces the disease-promoting effects of diabetes and Syndrome X. Most importantly, research has shown that this nutrient can prevent coronary heart disease, one of the key diseases caused by Syndrome X.[20] It may also play a role in lowering the risk of breast cancer, as free radical damage to DNA is one of the chief underlying causes of cancer.

To help protect against Syndrome X, diabetes, heart disease and breast cancer, 400 IU of natural (d-alpha) vitamin E daily should be sufficient. To help reverse these conditions, 400–800 IU of natural vitamin E could prove beneficial.

Vitamin C

Vitamin C helps protect against Syndrome X and its accompanying disorders by blocking many of the damaging effects of elevated glucose and insulin and reducing the free radical damage that contributes to heart disease, diabetes and cancer. For overall well-being and to increase your resistance to Syndrome X, take 1,000–2,000 mg of vitamin C daily. To help reverse Syndrome X, take 2,000–4,000 mg of vitamin C daily.

Chromium

An important mineral for the prevention and treatment of insulin resistance and Syndrome X, chromium helps insulin function more efficiently, aids fat loss and weight control and improves fat metabolism. Not only can it improve insulin function it can also lower cholesterol and decrease the risk of heart disease and high blood pressure. For the general prevention of Syndrome X, 200 mg of chromium picolinate daily should be sufficient. If you've got any of the conditions involved in Syndrome X, increase your supplement intake to 400–800 mg daily.

Zinc

Zinc plays a crucial role in glucose regulation and the proper function of insulin and weight control, while a zinc deficiency puts you at greater risk of Syndrome X. Optimal amounts of zinc vary among individuals, but 30 mg daily is a good dose for most women with PCOS.

Magnesium

Magnesium is necessary for the production and release of insulin. Magnesium supplementation is an important aid for people with glucose intolerance and insulin resistance. Magnesium also appears to protect against high blood pressure and cardiovascular disease. Magnesium is also essential for the proper functioning of the heart. Because magnesium helps insulin efficiency, virtually any woman with PCOS can benefit from a 400 mg daily magnesium dose.

Herbal remedies

To prevent insulin resistance and Syndrome X, herbs such as garlic, cinnamon, cloves and bay leaves could prove beneficial. To reverse insulin resistance and Syndrome X, silymarin or milk thistle supplements are often recommended. Other herbs that could prove beneficial if you've got Syndrome X include:

- Fenugreek (see page 200)
- Bitter melon (page 199)
- Gymnema sylvestre (page 200)
- Stevia (a plant extract eaten as an alternative to high-calorie sweeteners – researchers have found it to be good for reducing blood glucose levels[21]).

ASK YOUR DOCTOR

66 *Nothing can make more of a difference if you've got PCOS than a sympathetic doctor. It's the difference between feeling like a burden, as if you're somehow to blame for your problems and feeling understood, as a woman with a medical condition that can make losing weight hard and can affect the quality of your health and your life. I think the single most important thing for a woman who's got PCOS is to find a doctor who understands PCOS and is aware of the symptoms, risks and complications and the pros and cons of the various treatment options. So*

my advice to you if your doctor doesn't listen to you or won't consider treatment alternatives is to ditch him or her and find one who does listen and is willing to explore the options. 🙶

Linda, 41

There's no doubt that medications can play an important role in preventing and treating the symptoms of PCOS and the long-term health risks associated with them. However, PCOS is a lifelong condition that responds better when you take your health into your own hands. This doesn't mean ignoring your doctor's advice if medication is recommended. It's important to listen to what your doctor has to say, as in some cases medication can save lives – but make sure you understand the reasons why you're being offered a particular course of treatment, the implications of starting a course of treatment, and the options open to you.

Ask your doctor lots of questions. Are there alternatives you can explore? What are the side-effects? Is this the only way? Find out specifically how the drugs you're being prescribed actually work within your system to influence your condition. Ask for the name of the drug and the trade name to be written down for you so you can do some of your own research.

Don't feel pressured to make a decision straight away, and don't be shy about asking for a second opinion. Try to get advice and support from other women with PCOS and weigh up the positives and negatives so you can make an informed decision. With your future health and well-being at stake this is, after all, a very important decision. Give it the time and attention it deserves.

REFERENCES

1.   Cranner, P. *et al.*, 'Fifteen-year mortality in Coronary Drug Project patients: long-term benefit with niacin', *J Am Coll Cardiol* 1986 Dec; 8 (6): 1245–55
2.   Wagh, A. *et al.*, 'Treatment of metabolic syndrome', *Expert Rev Cardiovasc Ther* 2004 Mar; 2 (2): 213–28

3. Zimmermann, C. *et al.*, 'L-arginine-mediated vasoreactivity in patients with a risk of stroke', *Cerebrovasc Dis* 2004; 17 (2–3): 128–33

4. Digiesi, A. *et al.*, 'Coenzyme Q10 in essential hypertension', *Mol Aspects Med* 1994; 15 Suppl: s257–63

5. Mennen, L. I. *et al.*, 'Consumption of foods rich in flavonoids is related to a decreased cardiovascular risk in apparently healthy French women', *J Nutr* 2004 Apr; 134 (4): 923–6

6. Takata, A. *et al.*, 'Total care for patients with metabolic syndrome', *Nippon Rinsho* 2004 Jun; 62 (6): 1164–9

7. Brace, L. M. *et al.*, 'Cardiovascular benefits of garlic (Allium sativum L)', *J Cardiovasc Nurs* 2002 Jul; 16 (4): 33–49

8. Wilburn, A. J. *et al.*, 'The natural treatment of hypertension', *J Clin Hypertens* (Greenwich) 2004 May; 6 (5): 242–4

9. Ibid.

10. Rigelsky, J. M. *et al.*, 'Hawthorn: pharmacology and therapeutic uses', *Am J Health Syst Pharm* 2002 Mar 1; 59 (5): 417–22

11. Hahn, S. *et al.*, 'Metformin, an efficacious drug in the treatment of polycystic ovary syndrome', *Dtsch Med Wochenschr* 2004 May 7; 129 (19): 1059–64; Barbieri, R. L. *et al.*, 'Metformin for the treatment of the polycystic ovary syndrome', *Minerva Ginecol* 2004 Feb; 56 (1): 63–79

12. Dicter, N. *et al.*, 'Alpha-lipoic acid inhibits glycogen synthesis in rat soleus muscle via its oxidative activity and the uncoupling of mitochondria', *J Nutr* 2002 Oct; 132 (10): 3001

13. Kim, D. S. *et al.*, 'Chromium picolinate supplementation improves insulin sensitivity in Goto-Kakizaki diabetic rats', *J Trace Elem Med Biol* 2004; 17 (4): 243–7

14. Kely, G. S. *et al.*, 'Insulin resistance: lifestyle and nutritional interventions', *Altern Med Rev* 2000 Apr; 5 (2): 109–32

15. Mohan, V. *et al.*, 'Fenugreek and insulin resistance', *J Assoc Physicians India* 2001 Nov; 49: 1055–6

16. Baskaran, K. *et al.*, 'Antidiabetic effect of a leaf extract from Gymnema sylvestre in non-insulin-dependent diabetes mellitus patients', *J Ethnopharmacol* 1990 Oct; 30 (3): 295–300

17. Murakami, C. *et al.*, 'Screening of plant constituents for effect on glucose transport activity in Ehrlich ascites tumour cells', *Chem Pharm Bull (Tokyo)* 1993 Dec; 41 (12): 2129–31

18. Sanuncu, T. *et al.*, 'Sibutramine has a positive effect on clinical and metabolic parameters in obese patients with polycystic ovary syndrome', *Fertil Steril* 2003 Nov; 80 (5): 1199–204

19. Midaoui, A. E. *et al.*, 'Lipoic acid prevents hypertension, hyperglycemia, and

the increase in heart mitochondrial superoxide production', *Am J Hypertens* 2003 Mar; 16 (3): 173–9

20. Munteanu, A. *et al.*, 'Anti-atherosclerotic effects of vitamin E – myth or reality?', *J Cell Mol Med* 2004 Jan-Mar; 8 (1): 59–76
21. Curi, R., 'Effect of Stevia rebaudiana on glucose tolerance in normal adult humans', *Braz J Med Biol Res* 1986; 19: 771–4

16 Research Continues ...

We've looked at all the proven long-term health risks for us women with PCOS, and talked about the ways both you and your healthcare practitioners can tackle them now to help prevent them in the future. But in the history of PCOS, it seems science can lag behind what women with PCOS are talking to each other about all the time. So what about all those other problems that women in the PCOS communities wonder about? Are issues like an underactive thyroid, skin tags, pelvic pain, depression or lowered immunity all a direct risk of having PCOS? Are we more likely to get endometriosis, ovarian cysts and eating disorders? Or is it just the case that, as so many women have PCOS (thought to be one in 10 in the UK, US and Australia), some of us are bound to get other conditions as well by sheer chance? We've done some digging to find out, and this chapter is the result.

UNDERACTIVE THYROID (HYPOTHYROIDISM)

66 *At the age of 18 I was diagnosed with PCOS. I was put on the Pill to regulate my periods. Then in my early thirties I turned from an active mother of one to someone who barely had the energy to get up the stairs. My weight soared by nearly 40 pounds and I hated the way I looked. Emotionally I was all over the place. I'd lash out at my husband and son for very little reason. I couldn't concentrate at all and my work as a primary school teacher suffered. Parents' evening was a nightmare. I couldn't remember the names of the kids I'd taught for years. Not to*

mention the constant bouts of flu. When my periods stopped altogether I went to see my doctor, who diagnosed hypothyroidism. I wasn't shocked. To be honest I was at the point when I was just pleased to find out why I had been feeling so ill. I wasn't going crazy after all. 99

Isabelle, 34

Your thyroid is a butterfly-shaped gland located at the base of your neck. Although it weighs less than an ounce, the thyroid gland has an enormous effect on your health. All aspects of your metabolism, from the rate at which your heart beats to how quickly you burn calories, are regulated by thyroid hormones.

As long as your thyroid releases the proper amounts of these hormones, your system functions normally. But sometimes your thyroid doesn't produce enough hormones, upsetting the delicate balance of chemical reactions in your body. This condition is known as hypothyroidism. About 6 to 7 million Americans, mainly women over 40, have an underactive thyroid. Because hypothyroidism usually develops slowly, only about half of all cases are diagnosed early. At first, you may have few noticeable symptoms, or you may just feel tired and sluggish. But over time, untreated hypothyroidism can cause a number of health problems, such as recurring bouts of illness, obesity, high blood pressure, heart disease and diabetes.

Although anyone can develop hypothyroidism, it occurs mainly in women over 40, and the risk of developing the disorder increases if you're overweight, have irregular periods, high cholesterol and/or insulin resistance/diabetes. Sound familiar? Many of the symptoms and risk factors of hypothyroidism mirror those of PCOS, and this does seem to suggest that our risk for hypothyroidism is potentially higher than for a woman without PCOS. In fact, because the conditions can appear so similar, you may find that your doctor will want to rule out hypothyroidism before a definitive diagnosis of PCOS can be made.

Since all the hormonal systems in your body are interconnected, it's logical to assume that the hormonal havoc PCOS causes could trigger an imbalance in thyroid hormone production, or that an imbalance in thyroid hormones could trigger PCOS. And there do seem to be strong links between the two conditions, with similar symptoms, such as weight gain and irregular periods, and risk factors, such as high cholesterol and insulin resistance.

Although the likelihood of a connection between PCOS and hypothyroidism is strong, at present there just isn't enough evidence to point conclusively to this. Early research is, however, tentatively suggesting a possible connection.[1] PCOS expert and reflexologist Jacqui Garnier totally believes that there's a link. 'Reflexology is particularly helpful for women with PCOS,' she says, 'because of its ability to stimulate and rebalance the endocrine system, particularly the pituitary, hypothalamus and thyroid, and of course the ovaries. This in turn will help regulate the cycles, reduce excess production or inefficient amounts of particular hormones, as is typical with PCOS. The least women can expect is a regulation of the cycles when using reflexology. I have also found it helpful in encouraging more frequent ovulation. In fact, almost all my clients with PCOS – both overweight and underweight – also have a problem with their thyroids and there's no doubt in my mind of the connection.'

If you're feeling tired for no reason or have any of the other symptoms of hypothyroidism, such as poor concentration, cold hands and feet, low libido, mood swings, dry skin, hair loss, irregular periods, severe PMS, unexplained weight gain, headaches and constipation, go and see your doctor. If your cholesterol is high, talk to your doctor about whether hypothyroidism may be a cause. And if you're insulin resistant or have diabetes, talk to your doctor about the link with hypothyroidism, as low thyroid function is more frequently found in people with diabetes.

If hypothyroidism is diagnosed, the aim of any course of treatment is to normalize thyroid function and restore good health. Standard treatment for an underactive thyroid involves daily use of the synthetic thyroid hormone levothyroxine (Levothroid, Synthroid). This oral medication restores adequate hormone levels, shifting your body back into normal gear.

Soon after starting treatment, you'll notice that you're feeling less fatigued. The medication also gradually lowers cholesterol levels elevated by the disease, and may reverse any weight gain. Treatment with levothyroxine is usually for life.

Although most doctors recommend synthetic thyroxine, natural extracts containing thyroid hormone, derived from the thyroid glands of pigs, are also available. These products – Armour Desiccated Thyroid Hormone and Westhroid – more closely resemble natural thyroid hormones because they contain both thyroxine and tri-idothyronine. Synthetic thyroid medications contain thyroxine only.

Helping yourself

If your hypothyroidism is mild, medication may not be necessary if the underlying causes are considered and treated first. There are a number of possible causes of hypothyroidism including inflammation of the thyroid, the use of drugs that compromise thyroid function, and any illness, trauma or circumstance that depresses metabolism. This may be a transient reaction, lasting a few weeks, or a lifelong response causing irreversible thyroid collapse.

Iodine deficiency is also associated with thyroid problems. Iodine is a mineral found in seafood and it's essential for normal thyroid function. Certain foods reduce iodine function: Brussels sprouts, peaches, pears, spinach, turnips, soya, broccoli, cabbage, cauliflower, millet, maize, sweet corn, peanuts, almonds and walnuts. If you're suffering from thyroid deficiency you don't need to cut these out altogether, but you do need to limit your intake. It's also a good idea to avoid chloride and fluoride, found in toothpaste and tap water, as they can block receptors in the thyroid gland, resulting in reduced thyroid function. Helpful supplements include kelp, vitamin B complex, essential fatty acids, iron, vitamin A, C and E and the minerals selenium, manganese, copper, iron and zinc.

In common with PCOS there are often several factors involved in causing hypothyroidism. Weight gain, nutritional deficiencies, toxic overload and prolonged stress can all depress the entire endocrine system, including the thyroid. If you do find yourself in the difficult position of suffering from PCOS and hypothyroidism, talk to your doctor about the best treatment options. Whether medication is needed or not, symptoms can be greatly relieved by a healthy low GI diet (see page 80), regular exercise and weight loss if there's weight to lose.

Since PCOS and hypothyroidism are both hormonal disorders, the hormone-balancing diet and lifestyle changes recommended in the PCOS Protection Plan may be all that are needed to beat your symptoms, restore energy and good health. But always consult your doctor if your symptoms persist.

SKIN ABNORMALITIES

Skin abnormalities in women with PCOS can take a variety of forms. Skin 'tags' are tear-shaped pieces of skin usually found in the armpit or around the neck. They are often very small but can be as large as a raisin. They're usually painless, except for occasional irritation from rubbing by clothing, jewellery or other friction, and don't grow or change. Their origin is unknown but they're thought to be a symptom of insulin resistance, which many women with PCOS have, and can be removed by a physician. It isn't a good idea to try and remove or cut them off yourself, as this can cause inflammation and infection.

Apart from acne, another skin problem associated with PCOS is called *acanthosis nigricans*, a skin condition characterized by dark, thickened, velvety skin in body folds and creases. It usually develops over months or years, and most often affects the armpits, groin and neck. This disorder can be associated with diabetes and insulin resistance. In some cases, it may be inherited. Other causes include obesity, use of oral contraceptives and endocrine disorders. Although no research has been done, many women with PCOS do report suffering from this condition.

There's no effective treatment for acanthosis nigricans, but medications that may provide some improvement include insulin-lowering drugs such as metformin, or topical solutions such as Retin A alpha hydroxy acid and salicylic acid.

CHRONIC PELVIC PAIN

Some women with PCOS suffer from chronic pelvic pain. The pain can be steady or it can come and go. It could be a dull ache, a sharp pain or cramping. It can be an overall feeling of pressure or heaviness deep in your belly. You could have pain during intercourse, when you move your bowels or even when you plop into a chair. The pain may intensify after you stand for long periods and may be relieved when you lie down. The pain may be so bad that you miss work, can't sleep and can't exercise. The pain may vary from mild to severe, from annoying to downright disabling. One thing these various aches and pains have in common – besides being persistent – is that they occur in the area of your body referred to as your pelvic region – somewhere below your belly button and between your hips. If you were asked to locate your pain, you'd be more likely to sweep your hand over the entire area rather than point to one spot.

However you describe it, chronic pelvic pain is no stranger to women, whether you've got PCOS or not. One in seven women experience it and it accounts for 10 per cent of visits to gynaecologists. It's the reason behind at least 20 per cent of all laparoscopies – the viewing of your internal organs using a lighted tube inserted through a small incision in your abdomen – and for 12 to 16 per cent of hysterectomies (surgical removal of the uterus).

Determining what's causing your discomfort may be one of medicine's more puzzling and frustrating endeavours. It can be caused or triggered by any number of conditions, from endometriosis or ovarian cysts to fibroids. Although no research has been done, it's not difficult to see why many women with PCOS think there may be a link with this condition. In many cases, no physical cause may ever be discovered and as many as 61 per cent of women suffering from chronic pelvic pain never receive a specific diagnosis.

Women who are depressed, who are under excessive stress or who have been sexually or physically abused are more likely to experience chronic pelvic pain. That's because emotional distress can make any pain worse, possibly by causing you to tense your pelvic floor muscles or by causing chemical changes that affect your ability to cope with pain.

Treatment for chronic pelvic pain will depend on whether or not an exact cause, such as fibroids or endometriosis, is found. If no cause is found, treatment may include low-dose antidepressants, which may lessen pain, or psychotherapy, stress management or other relaxation techniques.

DIGESTIVE COMPLAINTS

66 *Some days my stomach just churns and churns and everything I eat, even something simple like a glass of apple juice, upsets it and I'm running for the restroom. Other times I'll suffer from constipation for days on end. Is this anything to do with my PCOS? Am I eating too much or too little fibre? Or perhaps dairy foods don't suit me? I wish I knew, as the constant turmoil inside is making me feel tired and irritable.* 99

Helen, 32

Many women with PCOS do complain of digestive problems, especially constipation and irritable bowel syndrome. So far research hasn't discovered why digestive complaints are common in women with PCOS, but it may have something to do with the slightly lowered metabolic rate that would make your digestive system that bit slower.

Certain drugs, such as antibiotics, can alleviate the malabsorption problems of digestive disorders, but dietary modification should be the first line of treatment. Healthy eating according to the Protection Plan diet guidelines, making sure you get enough fibre and drinking plenty of water are the best solutions for digestive complaints. Take your multivitamin, too, to make sure you're getting all your nutrients. Also watch out for food allergies and certain foods that trigger problems.

Lactose, found in milk and dairy products, is a common culprit; alcohol and tobacco can irritate the linings of the stomach and colon.

When an intestinal upset occurs, make your diet blander than usual. Stick to alkaline foods such as fruit and vegetables and avoid acid-forming foods such as meat, fish, eggs, cheese, grains, bread, flour, sugar, peas, beans, nuts, legumes, tea, coffee, alcohol and milk.

Research has also found that that people who practise stress management have fewer and less severe attacks, and that deep breathing exercises can help relieve digestive complaints (shallow breathing reduces the oxygen available for proper bowel function). Chewing your food well and taking time when you eat as well as avoiding food a few hours before bedtime can also help.

LOWERED IMMUNITY

66 *If someone has a cold at work or goes down with the flu I know it's only a matter of days, hours sometimes, before I start to go down with it, too. Is poor immunity somehow connected to my PCOS?* **99**

Linda, 44

Do you find that when a cold is doing the rounds you're the first to succumb? Or are you forever recovering from sore throats, coughs, colds and flu? You aren't alone. Many women with PCOS say that they get ill far more often than women without PCOS.

There could be an explanation for the lowered immunity many women with PCOS suffer from. Research has suggested a link between lowered immunity and menstrual irregularity. A study done at the University of Birmingham and published in the online journal *Genetics* has suggested that the high testosterone levels associated with PCOS could be caused by a fault in the way the body processes the stress hormone cortisol.[2] Cortisol, the active form of the hormone, can be turned into cortisone, the inactive form, by enzymes in the body. Researchers have found some women with PCOS don't have these enzymes. This means their bodies cannot process cortisol properly, which causes higher levels of testosterone to be produced. So it seems that we may not be able to deal with stress as effectively as women without PCOS. And it is generally accepted that people under stress are more prone to suffer infections due to a weakened immune system.

More research needs to be done, but simply knowing that your stress threshold may not be as strong as a woman who hasn't got PCOS can encourage you further to take steps to stress-proof your life. And what's the best way to do that? (as if you didn't know what we're going to say!). Stick to the advice in our Protection Plan. Eat healthy, nutritious food and exercise regularly to boost your immunity, and follow the stress management guidelines on pages 159–161.

CHRONIC FATIGUE

66 *It's always the morning after the night before for me. Trouble is there hasn't been a night before as I'm tucked up exhausted in bed by 9 p.m. most nights. However long I sleep I always wake up feeling tired, have a brief period of alertness in the morning and then get more and more tired as the day wears on. I used to think it was because I had PCOS but now that I've met other women with PCOS who are energetic and lead active, busy lives, can I still blame PCOS?* **99**

Lily, 30

Many women with PCOS complain of tiredness. Although fatigue or lack of energy isn't recognized as a symptom of PCOS, the hormonal fluctuations underlying the condition can also lead to difficulty getting a good night's sleep, so it's no wonder fatigue is an issue. And fatigue can be caused by a number of other things besides sleepless nights.

The hormonal imbalances you're experiencing when you've got PCOS can be a major factor in fatigue. Tiredness may also be a symptom of PCOS insulin problems and the higher than normal levels of oestrogen associated with the disorder. Dr Stephen Goldstein, associate professor of Obstetrics and Gynaecology at New York University's School of Medicine, says that research has shown that unopposed oestrogen (without progesterone to balance it) can be responsible for feelings of exhaustion and that sluggish, low-energy feeling.

If you're taking any medications to combat PCOS these can also be implicated in fatigue. It's important to mention your fatigue to your doctor and to find out if this is one of the known side-effects of your medication, and then discuss other medication options.

Besides sleeplessness, drugs and hormonal imbalance, there are other factors that can contribute to fatigue. The constant mental anxiety that occurs when unpleasant symptoms of PCOS are on your mind can itself be fatiguing. Without a doubt there are numerous connections between fatigue and PCOS, but the question is, does all this put us at risk of longer-term problems such as ME (also known as chronic fatigue syndrome)?

The simple answer is we don't know, but as the potential is there it makes sense to take steps to get rid of feelings of tiredness before they develop into something more serious.

Treating PCOS and managing it with self-help measures, such as diet, exercise, stress management and relaxation routines, as recommended in the Protection Plan, can certainly help you beat fatigue. If you find it hard to get a good night's sleep, the tips on pages 156–157 will be especially useful. And don't forget that fatigue may not be directly related to PCOS at all. It's important to have regular checks to rule out certain possibilities like nutritional deficiencies, allergies, food intolerances and anaemia.

ENDOMETRIOSIS

66*I've got PCOS and endometriosis and I'm convinced that the two are linked. I'm also convinced that PCOS makes symptoms of endometriosis more painful and even harder to cope with.*99

Annie, 37

Endometriosis is a common and often painful disorder of the female reproductive system. In this condition, a specialized type of tissue that normally lines the inside of your uterus (the endometrium) becomes implanted *outside* your uterus, most commonly on your fallopian tubes, ovaries or the tissue lining your pelvis. Rarely, endometrial tissue may spread beyond the pelvic region.

During your menstrual cycle, hormones signal the lining of your uterus to thicken to prepare for possible pregnancy. If a pregnancy doesn't occur, your hormone levels decrease, causing the thickened lining of your uterus to shed. This results in bleeding that exits your body through the vagina – your monthly period. When endometrial tissue is located in other parts of your body, it continues to act in its normal way: it thickens, breaks down and bleeds each month as your hormone levels rise and fall. However, because there's nowhere for the blood from this mislocated tissue to exit your body, it becomes trapped, and surrounding tissue can become irritated. Trapped blood may lead to the growth of cysts. Cysts, in turn, may form scar tissue and adhesions – abnormal tissue that binds organs together. This process can cause pain in the area of the misplaced tissue, usually the pelvis, especially during your period.

Endometriosis can also cause fertility problems. In fact, scars and adhesions on ovaries or fallopian tubes can prevent pregnancy.

It's not uncommon to see both PCOS and endometriosis in the same woman. Are the two conditions linked? Some PCOS experts believe that they are. 'It would seem logical,' says Dr Samuel Thatcher, 'that endometriosis would be more common in women with PCOS.' Thatcher lists PCOS as one of the risk factors for endometriosis, but at present no one has the definitive answer. What we do know is that sufferers of each share a common bond. Aside from being extremely common and with a genetic predisposition, both disorders are long term, affect lifestyle, lack a common cause or cure and are linked to hormone imbalance (typically excess amounts of oestrogen) – and it's this high level of oestrogen which often makes the symptoms of endometriosis worse for women who also have PCOS.

Endometriosis may improve for some women during pregnancy, when progesterone overtakes oestrogen and there are no periods. Medical treatments involve creating a state of 'pseudo pregnancy' or the menopause to limit the production of oestrogen; surgical treatments in severe cases can involve removal of the ovaries.

Both PCOS and endometriosis respond well to self-help measures, such as the healthy diet, regular exercise and stress management advice recommended in the Protection Plan, combined with the recommended care from your healthcare practitioner.

OVARIAN CYSTS

Polycystic ovary syndrome and ovarian cysts are often confused with one another, but it's important to point out that the cysts present in PCOS are not the same kind as those referred to as ovarian cysts. Ovarian cysts are found inside the ovary and they're usually single and larger than the cysts associated with PCOS. They can also be quite painful if they rupture or rotate, whereas the ring of smaller, more numerous cysts classic to PCOS are not typically noticed by the woman who has them.

Polycystic ovaries are thought to be caused by eggs that never leave the ovary because of the abnormal cycles experienced by women with PCOS. The egg follicles collect around the border of the ovary in a pattern commonly referred to as a string of pearls. Polycystic ovaries are a consequence rather than a cause of hormonal imbalance, and shouldn't be removed by surgery because, once the underlying hormonal imbalance is corrected, the cysts usually reduce in number. Ovarian cysts, on the other hand, grow to such a size that they interfere with ovarian function and in the great majority of cases they need to be removed surgically because they can carry the potential for ovarian cancer.

At present there isn't universal agreement on the cause of ovarian cancer, although, because the incidence of ovarian cancer seems to decrease in women who have had time off ovulation (either through pregnancy or the use of oral contraceptives), the theory of incessant ovulation as a risk factor has been suggested. Other theories name oestrogen as the culprit or suggest the involvement of androgens or progesterone. This could be bad news for PCOS sufferers, but on the other hand high levels of androgen can inhibit ovulation and protect against ovarian cancer. Some theories include exposure to toxins, but to date no one theory has received universal support and the general consensus is that there may be multiple causes of ovarian cancer.

So are women with PCOS more likely to get ovarian cysts? Again, the jury's still out. A 1996 study reported an increased risk of ovarian cancer among women with PCOS in a population-based, case-controlled study, but more recent research suggests that there simply isn't enough evidence.[3] So, although the possibility is there, the link is by no means established.

DEPRESSION

❝I do feel that I've had a lot of bad luck in my life. I was diagnosed with PCOS when I was 14 and missed out on all the teenage fun. I didn't have any friends. Not surprising really. I had bad acne, no waistline and felt I'd be fat and ugly for the rest of my life. All I could think was "Why me?" Things didn't get easier in my twenties. I just isolated myself more and more. Then when I was 28 I finally met a guy who liked me but I wouldn't let him near me because I was convinced I'd never be able to have children and he deserved better. Looking back, I can see that I was heading for a nervous breakdown. I'm still bitter about the way PCOS stole my youth.❞

Nina, 37

According to a 1990 World Health Organization study, depression is ranked as the fourth most deadly disease worldwide and is expected to be second only to heart disease by 2020.

Depression can manifest in physical symptoms such as headaches, stomach problems, insomnia, absence of periods, emotional symptoms such as sadness, emptiness, guilt and hopelessness, and behavioural changes such as memory loss, lack of libido, loss of concentration and withdrawal from social interactions.

Depression is typically associated with any chronic medical condition, and with many medications such as those used to treat high cholesterol and hypertension. Thyroid problems can cause depression, and a number of studies have linked abnormal cholesterol levels to depression. Another study reported that the incidence of depression was higher in people who suffered from chronic headaches. Many studies also indicate that depression is more likely to affect women than men, and this may be linked to the hormonal fluctuations associated with menstruation, childbirth and the menopause.[4]

So, is depression more common in women with PCOS? One study presented at the US PCOSA conference in 2000 suggested that it was specifically bi-polar disorder (lows followed by highs) that was linked with PCOS, but the jury is still out as to whether there's a direct link.

PCOS can be frightening, overwhelming and discouraging. Anxiety about appearance, grief about loss of control over family planning and anger at years of misdiagnosis are all common. When you add to that fears about elevated risk of life-threatening medical conditions in the future and the side-effects of medication, it can seem hopeless. Small wonder women can suffer depression as a side-effect of PCOS, or they may feel depressed because of PCOS-related difficulties. It can be tough to know which came first, the depression or the PCOS, but one thing is clear from PCOS research: PCOS can and does have a negative effect on mood, libido, and your sense of well-being.[5]

If you do feel low, often talking things through with people who care about you, with a counsellor or other women with PCOS can help. In severe cases of depression, prescription antidepressants are often used. There are no specific antidepressants used to treat women with POCS, and you may have to switch types before you find the one that works best for you.

In the absence of serious depression, self-help measures and changes in diet, environment and activity can help boost well-being and feelings of control. Some experts believe that regular exercise is as good as psychotherapy in helping elevate mood. If nutrition is poor our bodies are stressed and we are not able to respond well to the demands of daily life. Physical well-being is an important part of controlling our moods, and our attitude is important, too. A person with a negative attitude is more likely to feel depressed.

If self-help measures are not working, ask for help; this isn't sign of weakness but a sign that you're in control.

Chromium and depression

One study has found that nutritional supplementation with chromium in the form of chromium picolinate significantly improved carbohydrate cravings and other symptoms of depression. The results, which were presented at the 24th International Neuropsycho-pharmacology Congress (CINP) in Paris in June 2004, suggest that chromium picolinate may offer a new treatment option for depressed patients who find it difficult to stay on current prescription medication because of common, but often intolerable side-effects, such as sexual dysfunction and weight gain.[6] Other data from the study were released at a US National Institutes of Mental Health (NIMH) conference in Phoenix, Arizona, and builds on the beneficial effects of chromium picolinate reported in a recent pilot study published in the *Journal of Biological Psychiatry.*

Researchers believe that chromium's essential role as an insulin co-factor may be the biological link between chromium, carbohydrate cravings and depression. Insulin has effects on metabolic function that may affect serotonin levels in the brain. Impaired insulin function, which leads to poor glycaemic control, is linked to a number of health conditions including diabetes, where the incidence of depression is two times greater than in those who do not have diabetes. Numerous clinical studies (as reported in the June 2004 issue of *Food and Chemical Toxicology*) show that supplementation with chromium, in the form of chromium picolinate, is safe and helps improve insulin insensitivity and diabetes. As it may also play a role in alleviating depression, it may be of particular help to women with PCOS, insulin resistance and depression.

PCOS MOOD-BOOSTING TIPS

- Refocus negative thoughts to positive ones and talk positively to yourself. If you were disappointed today, tell yourself, 'It didn't happen today, but tomorrow is another day.'
- Stop negative thoughts.
- Plan to have some fun every day.
- Eat little and often and follow the Protection Plan diet guidelines.
- Make an effort to interact socially with people.
- Reach out to other women with PCOS – join a PCOS support group or PCOS website.
- Nurture yourself.
- Nurture your family and friends.
- Try different relaxation techniques every day (visualization, listening to music, a warm bath, prayer) and then choose a few that work best for you.
- Take time out for personal interests and hobbies.
- Listen to your body.
- Exercise for 20 to 30 minutes every day.

EATING DISORDERS

66 *When I was diagnosed with PCOS in my first year of college I was told that losing weight would ease my symptoms. I tried to lose weight and nothing worked so I simply stopped eating. I got so ill that I had to go to hospital.* 99

Lucy, 25

66 *I only have to look at a cake and I gain weight! Before I knew I had PCOS and that helped me explain it, I was paranoid about what I ate in case it made me even fatter. I still can't eat sweet things without feeling guilty, so I usually end up bingeing on a whole packet of biscuits or a whole cake instead of one slice, and then feel so bad I make myself throw up, I know it's stupid but I just can't help it.* 99

Stacey, 41

❝*I associate weight gain with being fat, hairy and unattractive. Losing weight improves my symptoms and it's easy for me to take things too far. I'm still afraid of eating normally and frequently binge, vomit and take laxatives to keep my weight down. Each time I say "Never again" but it keeps happening.* **❞**

Giselle, 34

Many women with PCOS feel that the condition has made them more vulnerable to eating disorders such as bulimia, or disordered eating patterns. A recent study suggested that PCOS does not *cause* eating disorders,[7] but since weight management problems are a common symptom of PCOS it's hardly surprising that research suggests that as many as 60 per cent of women with PCOS have eating problems like bulimia.[8] Even though medical opinion is divided, many PCOS experts such as Dr Helen Mason are convinced of the link. It's possible that episodes of starving and bingeing could trigger insulin metabolism problems and the symptoms of PCOS. It's also possible that the weight gain associated with PCOS increases the likelihood of eating disorders as a misguided attempt to lose weight. 'I'm just writing a paper for an eating disorder journal which will have a title like "Which comes first: PCOS or bulimia?" says Dr Mason. 'This shows that the link is not even really questioned now by many doctors and researchers.'

A woman's relationship to food is often very complicated, whether she has PCOS or not. But knowing that weight gain can make your symptoms worse, along with the fact that insulin resistance and a slower metabolism means you put on weight more easily, could make you more vulnerable to dysfunctional eating patterns.

Perhaps you've tried to control your weight to ease your symptoms and this has led to an eating disorder, like bulimia, or perhaps you haven't got a full-blown eating disorder but still have an unhealthy attitude toward food and are basing your happiness and sense of self-worth on your food choices.

It can be hard not to see your body and food as the enemies when you've got PCOS. Denying yourself food, then binge-eating or comfort eating, can give you a feeling of control over your life, your body and your emotions, even if that control makes you feel unwell and unhappy in the long term. And the relief that this feeling of control brings can be so powerful that it becomes addictive and starts a cycle of emotional eating that's hard to break.

It goes without saying that, apart from making you feel miserable and a slave to food, dysfunctional eating will make your PCOS symptoms worse. You won't be getting all the nutrients you need to balance your blood sugar and hormone levels, and this could disrupt the delicate insulin mechanism further and even trigger more symptoms. Weight loss will be even harder as you're confusing your metabolic rate and you'll also increase your risk of long-term health problems.

If you've been diagnosed with PCOS and have been or are starting to binge, diet or yo-yo diet, you need to tackle your disordered eating patterns before you tackle your PCOS. It's important that you seek support from your doctor, a counsellor, an eating disorder support group or a dietician. Key to your recovery will be building self-esteem, learning to separate negative feelings about yourself from food, and to pursue a healthy, not a thin, lifestyle which involves listening to your body and eating when you're hungry as opposed to eating for emotional, social or other reasons. For more advice on healing your relationship with food, see page 130.

Warning: If your eating patterns are so out of control that the quality of your life is being affected, it's important that you seek medical advice immediately.

CELLULITE

    66 *The media goes into a frenzy whenever a celebrity commits the cardinal sin of exposing cellulite. I guess it's supposed to make us feel better, seeing the rich, young and famous with orange peel thighs, but it just depresses me. The more fuss people make about cellulite, the more gross it*

seems and the more women like me with PCOS and enough cellulite for five women, suffer. **99**

Rebecca, 35

Although it's often seen as a merely cosmetic concern, many experts believe that cellulite occurs when circulation is sluggish and trapped toxins and waste products build up in the body. Its superficial appearance can vary widely. Some women develop a fairly consistent orange peel effect, while others have irregular lumps, and sometimes cellulite is barely noticeable because that person's skin is well toned.

Female hormones programme cellulite to collect mainly around the hips and thighs where fat is concentrated in readiness for childbirth. As high levels of unwanted oestrogen are associated with PCOS, the big question is: are our bodies more programmed to hold on to toxins, and more likely to get cellulite than women without PCOS?

PCOS is associated with hormonal disruption and, although no studies have been done, it's easy to see why some experts believe that cellulite is more likely in women with PCOS. Contrary to popular belief, female hormones don't cause cellulite – although they do assist its progress. Hormones determine the size, shape and distribution of fat cells, and it seems you're more likely to get cellulite at times of hormonal disruption such as puberty, pregnancy and the menopause. Stress, poor diet, bad posture, poor circulation and a sedentary lifestyle are also thought to contribute to hormonal disruption and the formation of cellulite.

So what can you do? How do you stop your circulation becoming sluggish and how do you get rid of all the other factors that increase your propensity to develop cellulite? It's a question of boosting your circulation, bringing your body back into balance and keeping it that way. The answer is simple – the Protection Plan. Diet, exercise, stress reduction and detoxing all need to be addressed. So the good news is that if you're starting or working with the Protection Plan, you'll inevitably reduce any cellulite you might have and/or prevent new cellulite forming – what a great side-effect!

HEADACHES

Migraine headaches are generally described as a severe pain on one or both sides of the head, an upset stomach and problems with vision. An attack can last a few hours or up to one or two pain-wracked days. There are some indications that women with PCOS may be predisposed to migraines.

Many factors can trigger migraine headaches; identifying them is an important part of treatment. A headache diary used over a three-month period can be used to identify your triggers. You may find that a particular food, such as chocolate, coffee, spinach, onions, beans, cabbage, alcohol, cheese, eggs, red meat, pasta or foods with MSG (monosodium glutamate) triggers an attack. You may find that certain activities, such as exercise or constrictive clothing, or loud noises or the weather, can trigger your migraines, or that they seem to be related to muscle aches and pains. You may find that the ten or so days before your period is the most likely time for you to experience migraine.

Many women with PCOS say that they suffer from migraine headaches. It's likely that these could be linked to the response of your central nervous system to the hormonal fluctuations associated with the condition. But even though a connection is possible, so far no studies have been done to explore the relationship directly.

If your headaches are so severe that they're destroying the quality of your life, see your doctor to discuss your options. In less severe cases the best way to prevent and control migraine headaches is to take an aspirin at the start of an attack to raise your tolerance to the pain, eliminate foods and/or drinks from your diet which may trigger an attack, eat little and often to keep blood sugar stable (as low blood sugar can cause dilation of the blood vessels to the head) and exercise regularly (it's believed that regular exercise can lessen the severity and occurrence of migraines). Stress management is also important, as stress and muscle tension can trigger an attack.

A number of alternative therapies have achieved some success for women with migraines. Massage can enhance circulation and relax the muscles. Acupuncture and aromatherapy may also be helpful, as may yoga and t'ai chi.

THE BOTTOM LINE

Other conditions that may be affected by or linked to PCOS include:

- asthma – it's possible that oestrogen can worsen asthma
- fibroids – there's no doubt fibroids are related to oestrogen levels
- autoimmune disease and conditions which have an immunological basis such as Crohn's disease, arthritis, lupus and others.

There may even be more possible connections than those listed in this chapter, as no part of your body or disease process is immune from the effects of your hormones, and therefore could be connected to or affected by PCOS.

There's still so much to learn about PCOS, and because so little is known with absolute certainty it's important that you and your doctor play 'medical detective' as far as your PCOS and health and well-being are concerned. As new studies are completed and women with PCOS continue talking and gathering their own evidence, it's never been more important to stay informed, keep your eyes open to potential links and never dismiss the possibility of a connection between PCOS and other conditions.

REFERENCES

1. Bagavando, P. *et al.*, 'Transient induction of polycystic ovary-like syndrome in immature hypothyroid rats', *Proc Soc Exp Biol Med* 1998 Oct; 219 (1): 77–84
2. Gallinelli, I. *et al.*, 'Autonomic and neuroendocrine responses to stress in patients with functional hypothalamic secondary amenorrhea', *Fertil Steril* 2000 Apr; 73 (4): 812–6
3. Balen, A. *et al.*, *Hum Reprod Update* 2001 Nov-Dec; 7 (6): 522–5

4. Payne, J. L. *et al.*, 'The role of estrogen in mood disorders in women', *Int Rev Psychiatry* 2003 Aug; 15 (3): 280–90

5. Coffey, S. *et al.*, 'The effect of polycystic ovary syndrome on health-related quality of life', *Gynecol Endocrinol* 2003 Oct; 17 (5): 379–86; Elsenbruch, S. *et al.*, 'Quality of life, psychosocial well-being, and sexual satisfaction in women with polycystic ovary syndrome', *J Clin Endocrinol Metab* 2003 Dec; 88 (12): 5801–7; Rasgon, N. L. *et al.*, 'Depression in women with polycystic ovary syndrome: clinical and biochemical correlates', *J Affect Disord* 2003 May; 74 (3): 299–304; McIntyre, R. S. *et al.*, 'Valproate, bipolar disorder and polycystic ovarian syndrome', *Bipolar Disord* 2003 Feb; 5 (1): 28–35

6. Davidson, J. *et al.*, 'Effectiveness of chromium in atypical depression: a placebo-controlled trial', *Biol Psychiatry* 2003 Feb 1; 53 (3): 261–4

7. Michelmore, M. F. *et al.*, 'Polycystic ovaries and eating disorders: Are they related?', *Hum Reprod* 2001 Apr; 16 (4): 765–9

8. Jahanfar, S. *et al.*, 'Bulimia nervosa and polycystic ovary syndrome', *Gynecol Endocrinol* 1995 Jun; 9 (2): 113–17; McCluskey, S. *et al.*, 'Polycystic ovary syndrome and bulimia', *Fertil Steril* 1991 Feb; 55 (2): 287–91

17 Looking Ahead

PCOS is one of the most common hormonal disorder in women. Finally, after years of neglect and misdiagnosis, medical experts are at long last giving PCOS the attention it deserves. An extraordinary amount of research is currently being done to find out more about PCOS, and countless studies and research projects are underway.

Now that PCOS is more easily recognized and diagnosed, and the links between insulin and PCOS have been established, you can expect a continuing increase in the study of PCOS symptoms and their short- and long-term health effects. This can only be good news if you've got PCOS.

With all that we're learning about PCOS, there's light at the end of the tunnel and we can look ahead to greater awareness, understanding and better treatment options. But we aren't there yet. Many doctors are still not sufficiently enlightened about PCOS to be able to make a diagnosis readily and offer the best course of treatment, and many women still put their health at risk by ignoring symptoms such as facial hair, acne and irregular periods because they aren't aware of PCOS.

So what, apart from recommending this book and joining and/or volunteering to help a PCOS support group with its publicity, can you do to increase awareness of PCOS and its long-term health risks?

RESEARCH STUDIES AND CLINICAL TRIALS

"*I've always been interested in medical research. I'm a nurse and love my job, and as soon as I was diagnosed it was natural for me to want to*

*know more about what research was being done on PCOS. I asked around
at the hospital where I work and was put in touch with a researcher who
was conducting a study about PCOS and diet. I had no hesitations about
signing up for the study. It only lasted a few months and all I had to do
was write down everything I ate and record my PCOS symptoms. I really
feel good about being part of something that could, one day, help other
women with PCOS. I'd like to give talks at conferences and in medical
schools, not just about PCOS but about how other women can get involved
in cutting-edge research that one day could make all the difference.*

Sonia, 27

You can get involved in the future of PCOS by participating in research
studies and clinical trials. If you've got a strong interest in research of
your own condition, clinical trials can be very interesting and helpful
for yourself and potentially for other women with PCOS.

If you're interested in getting involved in a research study or clinical trial, first ask your doctor about any research being conducted in
your area. You can also contact your local medical school or teaching
hospital. Most typically it's the gynaecology or endocrinology departments that are interested in PCOS research. Sometimes a study
requires that you live close to the research centre, but some
research studies are just trying to gather information and will interview women nationwide. They'll simply have you complete a telephone
interview.

For women with PCOS who live in the UK, after consulting with
your doctor the PCOS support group Verity is a good first port of call,
as some clinical trials advertise there. You may also want to send a
stamped addressed envelope to PCOS expert Adam Balen, Professor of
Reproductive Medicine and Surgery, Clarendon Wing, Leeds General
Infirmary, Leeds LS2 9NS.

If you live in the US you can find out about national studies by
contacting PCOS-specific clinical trials listed on PCOS websites such
as PCOSA and Soulcysters. You can also find out about national studies
by contacting the National Institutes of Health in Maryland. This

Government-funded health research institute provides a website (www.clinicaltrials.gov) that identifies health-related research studies. (This site also lists information about clinical trials that are no longer recruiting.) You can also search the Center Watch site by condition as this lists, by conditions, clinical trials taking place all over the US (www.centerwatch.com).

Before taking part in a clinical trial, make sure both the researcher and the study site are reputable and have a good history of conducting clinical trials. Make sure, too, that you fit the requirements. For example, some studies will require women who are trying to get pregnant, so if a baby isn't on the agenda for you, don't apply. It's also important that you know what commitment you need to make and what expenses will be paid if travel is involved. Perhaps most important of all, you need to know what the purpose of the trial is. What is it trying to accomplish or find out? For example, is it to study the effectiveness of a certain medication? To try to determine how certain foods affect PCOS? To determine whether PCOS runs in families? Make sure you're comfortable with the goals of the trial, and if drugs are to be tested that you're aware of the side-effects. You should always be asked to sign a consent form if you want to take part in a trial, and this form should explain all the details of the trial and tell you exactly what you can expect. You should be given the opportunity to have all your questions about the trial answered – if there's anything that's unclear, don't sign the consent form. Have your doctor review the consent form and go over it with you. Finally, you need to know what's going to happen when the trial is completed and how you'll hear about the results.

Research on PCOS and clinical trials addressing PCOS are taking place in many countries all over the world, and the information they provide can help us feel more in control of our condition and the treatment options available. Some of the topics currently under study through clinical trials are:

• how PCOS affects moods

- PCOS and teenagers
- the influence of PCOS on the risk of developing heart disease and cancer
- experimental medications to manage PCOS-related symptoms
- PCOS and genetics
- the connection between PCOS and insulin resistance
- PCOS and sleep disordered breathing
- PCOS and menopause.

Information on all the above and other PCOS studies can be found on the clinical trial websites.

Getting involved in a clinical trial will involve time, commitment and dedication, but for many of the women with PCOS we have spoken to, getting involved gave them a great deal of satisfaction in knowing that they might be helping other women with PCOS.

If clinical trials aren't right for you, simply monitoring and being aware of what's on the horizon for treatment will arm you with more knowledge about what to discuss with your doctor when it comes to treating your symptoms.

Yes, there's a lot we don't know about PCOS, but the good news is we are learning more and more each day. There are more treatment options and self-help recommendations available than ever before. And because of the now accepted link of PCOS to insulin resistance and potential diabetes, you can rest assured that PCOS will never be ignored by the medical community again.

As the years go by and research goes on, there's no doubt more and more women will be able to deal with PCOS better and better, reclaiming their health and their lives.

YOUR FUTURE

If your symptoms are simply inconvenient and occasionally embarrass-ing, it can be tempting to ignore them. If you take only one thing away with you from this book, we hope it's this: PCOS symptoms, however mild, shouldn't be ignored.

As we've stressed throughout, regardless of whether your symptoms are mild or severe, the long-term health risks of PCOS are real. It's vital that you pay attention to your symptoms and the risk they pose to your future health, well-being and quality of life. PCOS offers you an opportunity to take the steps necessary to prevent diabetes, obesity, high blood pressure, Syndrome X, heart disease and perhaps even cancer. Seen in this light, PCOS is a gift, an early warning system other women don't have, so try not to waste this opportunity.

66*At the age of 12 I developed a dark patch of skin on my inner thigh. I hadn't noticed it before. My periods had started the year before but my cycles were irregular from the start. By age 16 I was bleeding for weeks instead of the usual days and my mom took me to the doctor. He did a laparoscopic exam and found lots of little cysts on my ovaries. I was put on the birth control pill and then metformin at the age of 18 when I started to develop facial hair. From the beginning of my treatment my doctor urged me to change my diet and up my exercise levels, and now at the age of 26 not only is my PCOS under control but I've probably gained a lot by recognizing the problem at such a young age. By the time I'm ready, if I choose to have babies I'll be ahead of the fertility game. And healthy eating and exercise have become a part of my life, which means my risk for developing diabetes, heart disease and other things is much lower.*99

Tracy, 26

66*I always sort of knew something was wrong. My body always felt as if it had a mind of its own, not falling into the normal category, but I just ignored my symptoms for years thinking it was just one of those things. It was when I wanted to get pregnant and couldn't that I found out I had PCOS. My doctor mentioned the increased risk of heart disease and diabetes, but at the time I didn't really listen. It was only a year after the birth of my baby boy when my doctor wanted to discuss treatment* *options for my PCOS that his words came back to haunt me. My family has a history of diabetes and lots of heart disease. From that moment on I took my health seriously. My diet has changed completely and I feel 10 years younger. It makes me laugh to think that it took giving birth to get me to this point with my health.* 99

Linda, 32

66 *There isn't a history of diabetes or heart disease or even obesity in my family, but as soon as I found out that PCOS increases my risk I decided to take charge of my health. There's at least one positive in a PCOS diagnosis – you get a warning, a chance to turn things around – which is something other women don't have. If there are things I can do to ease PCOS and increase my chances of a long and healthy life, I'd be a fool not to do them.* 99

Sonia, 26

66*PCOS is so hard to deal with. Your friends and family have never heard of it – you say you've got it and people's eyes glaze over. It's only when I relate it to diabetes that I get more understanding. I've done my research and, now I know the risks, I can do something about them. But what about all the women out there who go to see their doctor with a vague set of problems and are told to go home and take a nap? I'd like to see PCOS more out in the open so that women and girls with symptoms can go find out what they can do to get their bodies to function normally and increase their chances of good health now and in the years ahead.* 99

Jenna, 40

We never thought we'd say this, but both of us are grateful to PCOS for encouraging us to take charge of our health and take the steps necessary to prevent future complications. What we wanted to do in this book was to give you the information and guidance you need to maintain and, if necessary, restore your health and lower the odds against serious illness. We hope you'll use it to build a healthy, happy future for yourself.

Part Four
PCOS-Friendly Recipes

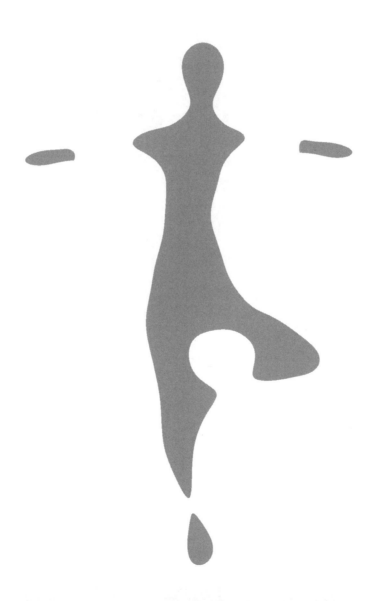

Cookery experts Amy Kashiwa Allsop and Victoria Bressette-Rebb have created some PCOS-friendly recipes that are good for you and delicious as well. If you'd like to learn more about Amy and Victoria's recipes, you can e-mail them at: amyallsop_uk@yahoo.com

---

Note

Some of these recipes contain red meat and dairy products. No, we haven't made a mistake! Reducing your intake of saturated fats doesn't mean you need to avoid red meat and dairy products entirely. As long as you choose lean cuts of red meat you can still include it in moderation (say once or twice a week) as part of your healthy diet.

If you choose not to eat red meat, legumes and tofu are good alternatives as they provide the protein, iron and zinc found in red meat. If you're vegetarian, replace the chicken stock in the soups with vegetable stock.

As long as dairy foods are replaced with reduced-fat varieties, you will keep your saturated fat intake right down. (Alternatively you could choose calcium-fortified soy products such as soy milk.)

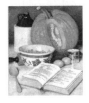 **STARTERS**

Guacamole dip

2 ripe Haas avocados
2 ripe tomatoes, de-seeded and chopped
2 oz/55 g onion, chopped
½ lime, juiced (about 1 tbs)
2 cloves garlic, minced
2 tbs chopped cilantro
sea salt (about ½ a tsp)

Halve and pit the avocados and place them in a mixing bowl. Chop the tomatoes and onion and add to avocado. Add lime juice, garlic, cilantro and sea salt to taste. Mash together with a fork and serve with fresh-cut vegetables, toasted pitta strips, fajitas or chilli.

Hummus

(Courtesy of Nahla Gholam of Mediterranean Specialties in Bellingham, WA)

1 tin chickpeas, or 6 oz/170 g boiled chickpeas
4 oz/115 g tahini
1 clove garlic
2 fl oz/60 ml lemon juice
Garnish: fresh parsley, 6–8 chickpeas, paprika, olive oil

Boil the chickpeas in enough water to cover them for 5 minutes. (If using chickpeas from a tin, rinse first and then boil in fresh water.) Place all ingredients in a food processor (saving 6–8 chickpeas for garnish) and puree for 5 minutes until the hummus is soft and creamy. Spread the hummus in a shallow serving dish and garnish with parsley leaves, chickpeas and paprika; drizzle with olive oil. Serve with pitta wedges, toasted pitta strips, olives, pickles and fresh vegetables.

Tabouleh

(Courtesy of Nahla Gholam of Mediterranean Specialties in Bellingham, WA)

2 oz/55 g parsley
5 stems fresh mint
4½ oz/135 g tomatoes
2 oz/55 g shallots
1 tbs fine bulgur (fine grind)
5 tbs extra virgin olive oil

2 fl oz/60 ml lemon juice
pinch salt, fresh pepper to taste
¼ tsp allspice

Rinse the parsley, mint, tomatoes and shallots. Let them air-dry overnight on a cotton tea towel or use a vegetable spinner to dry. (This is very effective.) First, chop the parsley and the shallots. Second, dice tomatoes into tiny squares (similar to salsa) and finely chop the mint and put into the centre of the diced tomatoes. Mix all of the ingredients in a salad bowl (except olive oil, lemon juice, salt, pepper and allspice) and place in the refrigerator for at least 2 hours until the bulgur is soaked. When ready to serve, add the olive oil, lemon juice, salt, pepper and allspice. Garnish with tomatoes and serve with cabbage or romaine lettuce hearts.

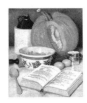 # SOUPS

Minestrone with chickpeas

4 oz/115 g chopped aubergine
4 oz/115 g chopped courgettes
5 oz/140 g chopped swede
2 oz/55 g chopped red bell pepper
2 oz/55 g chopped onion
1 garlic clove, minced
2 14-oz/395-g tins vegetable broth
1 28-oz/795-g tin diced tomatoes, undrained
1 bay leaf
1 tbs chopped fresh parsley

1 tbs pesto
1 tbs chopped fresh oregano
¼ tsp freshly ground black pepper
2 15-oz/425-g tins chickpeas, rinsed and drained
4 oz/115 g chopped spinach

Heat a large saucepan over medium-high heat. Coat pan with cooking spray. Add aubergines, courgettes, swede, red pepper, onion and garlic. Sauté 4 minutes or until the onion is tender. Stir in the broth, tomatoes and bay leaf; bring to a boil. Reduce heat and simmer 15 minutes. Discard bay leaf. Add parsley, pesto, oregano, black pepper and chickpeas; cook 5 minutes or until thoroughly heated. Stir in spinach; serve immediately.

Pork and green chilli soup with lettuce and cilantro

1 tbs canola oil
7 oz/200 g sweetcorn
2 oz/55 g chopped onion
8 oz/225 g diced pork, either raw or cooked
1 tin (4 oz/115 g) green chillies
1 tsp cumin
1 tsp oregano
1 tsp minced garlic
1 bay leaf
cayenne pepper to taste
1 tin (15 oz/425 g) diced tomatoes with their juice
16 fl oz/450 ml chicken broth
salt and pepper to taste

Garnish
6 oz/170 g shredded lettuce
2 oz/55 g chopped onion
1 oz/30 g chopped cilantro leaves
4 oz/115 g light sour cream (optional)

Heat oil in a large pot. Add sweetcorn and sauté over medium-high heat until brown. Stir in onion, pork, chillies, cumin, oregano, garlic, bay leaf and cayenne. Sauté until pork browns and begins to stick to the bottom of the pan.

Add the tomatoes and broth and bring to a boil. Reduce heat, cover and simmer for 30 minutes. Season with salt, if needed, and pepper; simmer for 30 minutes longer.

Serve in bowls and top with shredded lettuce, chopped onion, cilantro and sour cream, if desired.

Pumpkin soup

1½ tbs olive oil
4 oz/115 g onions, chopped
1 large clove garlic, minced
1 tsp curry powder
1/8 tsp ground coriander
1/8 tsp crushed red pepper
24 fl oz/675 ml (low-sodium) chicken broth. Vegetable broth can also be used.
10 oz/285 g pureed cooked pumpkin or tinned pumpkin puree
8 fl oz/225 ml low-fat milk

Sauté onions and garlic in olive oil. Add curry, salt, coriander and red pepper. Cook together several minutes. Add broth and boil gently for 20 minutes. Stir in pumpkin and milk. Cook 5 minutes. Puree to blend.

Chicken barley soup

1 medium onion, chopped
1 garlic clove, minced
1 tbs olive or vegetable oil
24 fl oz/675 ml water
1 15-oz/425 g tin whole-kernel sweetcorn, drained

1 15-oz/425-g tin black beans, rinsed and drained
1 15-oz/425-g tin tomato sauce
1 14½-oz/410-g tin diced tomatoes, undrained
1 14½-oz/410-g tin chicken broth
3½ oz/100 g medium pearl barley
1 4-oz/115-g tin chopped green chillies
1 tbs chilli powder
½ to 1 tsp ground cumin
1½ lb/680 g cubed cooked chicken

In a Dutch oven or soup kettle, sauté onion and garlic in oil until tender. Add the water, sweetcorn, black beans, tomato sauce, diced tomatoes, chicken broth, pearl barley, green chillies, chilli powder and ground cumin. Bring to a boil. Reduce heat; cover and simmer for 45 minutes. Stir in the chicken; cook 15 minutes longer or until chicken is heated through and barley is tender.

Three P soup

1½ lb/680 g yams or sweet potatoes
1 tbs low-fat butter
2 tbs minced shallot or onion
10 oz/285 g thick pumpkin puree, tinned or homemade
64 fl oz/1,820 ml (1 litre 820 ml) chicken broth, tinned or homemade
9 oz/255 g smooth peanut butter
2 tsp coarse-grain mustard
½ tsp nutmeg
sea salt
freshly ground white or black pepper
snipped chives (optional, for garnish)

Preheat oven to 350°F/180°C/Gas Mark 4. Bake yams on a baking sheet for 1 hour or until soft. Let cool and peel. Discard peels and process pulp in food processor. Measure out 10 oz/285 g and set aside. Refrigerate leftovers.

In a large, heavy-bottomed pot, melt butter over medium heat. Add shallots or onion and sauté for 2 minutes. Add the 10 oz/285 g of potatoes and the pumpkin puree. Alternately add broth and peanut butter, stirring the mixture after each addition until the soup is smooth. Over a medium heat, bring the soup almost to a boil, stirring often. Reduce heat and simmer for 25 minutes, stirring occasionally. Stir in mustard, nutmeg, salt and pepper. Garnish with chives.

Chickpea soup

6 fl oz/170 ml chicken broth
2 carrots, thinly sliced
3 cloves garlic, minced
½ tsp dried sage
¼ tsp pepper
6 fl oz/170 ml water
14 oz/395 g cooked or tinned chickpeas
4 oz/115 g packed, torn spinach or watercress leaves

Bring the broth to a boil over moderate heat. Add the carrots, garlic, sage and pepper, and cook for 5 minutes or until the carrots are tender. Add the water and chickpeas, and return to boil. Reduce to simmer, cover and cook for 7 minutes. Stir in greens and cook for 1 minute.

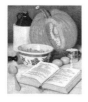 # MAIN DISHES

Rosemary-garlic pork

1 pork loin
3 cloves garlic, sliced
1 tbs of water

1 tsp olive oil
¼ tsp salt and pepper
10–12 fresh rosemary sprigs

Trim fat from pork loin. Make ½-inch slits in the pork and insert garlic into the holes.

Combine water, oil, salt and pepper. Rub the pork surface with the oil mixture and wrap in foil, adding the rosemary sprigs lengthwise inside around the pork loin. Cook at 400°F/200°C/Gas Mark 6 for 30 minutes or until pork is done.

Apple cranberry chutney

2 medium Golden Delicious apples, cored and cubed
2 tsp sugar
4 fl oz/115 ml red wine
2 tbs apple cider vinegar
¾ tsp ground ginger
⅛ tsp ground cloves
1 oz/30 g dried cranberries or raisins

Place apple cubes in a small frying pan with remaining ingredients. Bring to a simmer on medium-high heat. Lower heat to medium and cook gently until sauce begins to thicken (about 5 minutes). Serve with pork roast.

Chicken Yakitori skewers

3 large chicken breasts, cubed
mushrooms and cubed eggplant (optional)

Place cubes in marinade (see below) for 1 hour at room temperature. Meanwhile, if using bamboo skewers, soak in water to prevent from burning on grill.

Marinade
3 fl oz/90 ml dry sherry
3 tbs soy sauce (reduced sodium if preferred)
3 tbs sesame oil
1½ tsp grated fresh ginger

Remove skewer from marinade and grill or broil until cooked throughout (about 2 minutes each side). Roll in sesame seeds and serve. This
is a good appetizer; can be served at room temperature.

Bulkogi (Korean barbecue) marinade

1 lb/455 g chicken breasts cut into cubes
Marinate chicken for at least 30 minutes prior to cooking.

Marinade
2 tbs sesame seeds
3 fl oz/90 ml soy sauce
1 tbs sugar
2 cloves garlic, minced
2 shallots, chopped
¼ tsp black pepper
1 oz/30 g chopped green pepper
2 fl oz/60 ml toasted sesame oil

Grill or broil the marinated chicken, turning occasionally until cooked
through. Serve with white or brown rice.

Chicken cooked in wine

1 3-inch piece of pork, all fat removed
1 medium onion
1 clove garlic
cooking spray
8 chicken thighs or 8 small chicken breasts

¼ tsp each: ground cloves, allspice, ginger, cinnamon, nutmeg
salt and pepper to taste
1 8-fl oz/225-ml glass of red wine
2 chicken bouillon cubes (or equivalent) dissolved in 16 fl oz/450 ml hot water
6 tbs flour dissolved in 8 fl oz/225 ml cold water

Chop pork, shallots and garlic in food processor. Spray a large (8-pint) saucepan with cooking spray and add pork and shallot mixture. Add chicken and sprinkle with spices and seasonings. Add wine and simmer over medium heat (covered) for 10 minutes. Add chicken broth, cover and simmer for 1–2 hours.

Meanwhile, in a large jam jar combine the flour and cold water and shake well. Gradually add flour/water mixture to chicken mixture to thicken. Stir well and heat until bubbly. Serve with cooked polenta or rice.

Salmon marinade

2 fl oz/60 ml orange juice
2 fl oz/60 ml soy sauce (low sodium if preferred)
2 tbs ketchup
2 tbs olive oil
2 tsp parsley
2 tsp lemon juice
½ tsp dried oregano
⅛ tsp ground black pepper
1 garlic clove, minced

Mix all ingredients in a bowl. Pour over salmon fillet or steaks and chill, up to 8 hours, before grilling.

Baked pork chops with rice

salt

pepper

4 pork chops

cooking spray

7 oz/200 g rice

1 tin low-sodium beef consommé or bouillon (16 fl oz/450 ml)

4 slices each: onion, tomato, green pepper

Sprinkle salt and pepper over each pork chop. Brown pork chops on both sides in a non-stick pan. Spray the bottom of an 8 × 10-inch casserole dish with cooking spray and put dry rice in the bottom, cover with beef consommé or bouillon and place pork chops on top. Place one slice of onion, tomato and green pepper on each pork chop. Cover with foil and cook at 350°F/180°C/Gas Mark 4 for 1 hour or until pork is done.

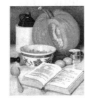 ## SALADS

Cabbage fruit salad

8 oz/225 g shredded cabbage

2 oranges, peeled and cut into bite-sized chunks (or tin of mandarin oranges)

6 oz/170 g seedless red grape halves

1 oz/30 g currants (or dried cranberries)

4 oz/115 g fat-free mayonnaise

2 fl oz/60 ml skim milk

1 tbs lemon juice

1 tbs sugar
1 oz/30 g chopped pecans, toasted

Toss cabbage and fruits. Combine mayonnaise, milk, lemon juice and sugar; cover and refrigerate. Just before serving, stir in pecans.

Sweetcorn and bean salad

2 15¼-oz/440-g tins whole kernel sweetcorn, drained
2 15-oz/425-g tins black beans, rinsed and drained
1 10-oz/285-g tin Mexican-style diced tomatoes and green chillies, undrained
3 oz/85 g thinly sliced shallots
3 fl oz/90 ml olive oil
3 fl oz/90 ml lime juice
1 tsp minced fresh cilantro or parsley
1 tsp ground cumin

Mix the sweetcorn, black beans, tomatoes, chillies and shallots in a large bowl. In another bowl, mix together the olive oil, lime juice, cilantro or parsley and cumin. Combine the two mixtures, cover and refrigerate for at least 2 hours. Serve with a slotted spoon.

Orzo salad

2 oz/55 g pine nuts, toasted
3 oz/85 g orzo pasta
6 oz/170 g frozen peas
3 oz/85 g marinated sun-dried tomatoes, chopped

Dressing
1 tbs Dijon mustard
2 oz/55 g minced shallots
2½ tbs balsamic vinegar
1 tsp pepper
3 fl oz/90 ml olive oil

To make dressing, whisk mustard, shallots, vinegar and pepper. Slowly add oil to thicken. Toss pine nuts in a frying pan over medium heat until toasted. Set aside. Cook orzo in salted, boiling water, until al dente. Do not overcook. Rinse with cold water and drain well. Rinse frozen peas in hot water to defrost. Pour dressing over orzo and mix in pine nuts, peas and sun-dried tomatoes. Serves 8.

Caprese salad

2 punnets cherry tomatoes, halved
4 oz/115 g part-skim mozzarella, cut into ¼-inch cubes
2 oz/55 g slivered green olives
½ oz/15 g chopped fresh basil
2 tbs balsamic vinegar
1 tbs olive oil

In a medium bowl, combine all of the ingredients.

Chicken-pistachio salad

2 oz/55 g shelled pistachio nuts, finely ground
pinch of salt
½ tsp freshly ground black pepper
4 boneless, skinless chicken breast halves
2 tbs olive oil
2 oz/55 g diced sweet white onion
¼ tsp salt
pinch of pepper
1 head romaine lettuce

Preheat the oven to 375°F/190°C/Gas Mark 5. Mix the nuts in a pie plate with the salt and pepper. Press the chicken into the nuts. Heat 1 tbs of the oil in a frying pan and cook the chicken, 2 minutes per side. Place in a baking dish and bake for 15 minutes or until a thermometer registers 160°F/75°C and the juices run clear.

Heat the remaining oil in a nonstick frying pan over high heat. Add the onion, salt and a pinch of pepper. Cook until the onion is browned.

Line four serving plates with lettuce. Slice the chicken breasts and arrange one breast on top of the lettuce on each plate. Serve with the dressing.

Dressing
1 tbs grated sweet white onion
1 large ripe avocado, pitted and peeled
3 tbs olive oil
3 tbs fresh lime juice
1 tbs water

Puree all ingredients in a blender.

Strawberry spinach salad

1 bag baby spinach
1 bag corn salad (or other greens of choice)
Few leaves of bib/butter lettuce, torn into bite-size pieces
About 12 sliced fresh strawberries

Dressing
Slight 2 fl oz/60 ml honey
2 fl oz/60 ml white vinegar
2 fl oz/60 ml oil (olive or sesame work well)
2 tbs sesame seeds or poppy seeds (or both)
⅛ tsp Worcestershire sauce
1 tbs minced onion

Mix together in a jar with a tight lid and shake well. Add to salad just before serving.

Orange-avocado salad

4 fl oz/115 ml vegetable oil
3 fl oz/90 ml white wine vinegar or cider vinegar

1 garlic clove, minced
2 tbs brown sugar
1 tsp curry powder
1 tsp soy sauce
30 oz/855 g torn red leaf lettuce
2 oz/55 g torn fresh spinach
1 11-oz/310-g tin mandarin oranges, drained
6 oz/170 g halved green grapes
2 oz/55 g slivered almonds, toasted
1 ripe avocado, peeled and sliced

In a jar with a tight-fitting lid, combine the oil, vinegar, garlic, brown sugar, curry powder and soy sauce; shake well.

In a large salad bowl, toss the lettuce, spinach, oranges, grapes and almonds. Add dressing and toss to coat. Garnish with avocado.

Chicken fajita salad

6 tbs vegetable oil, divided
4 fl oz/115 ml lime juice
2 tbs minced fresh parsley
2 garlic cloves, minced
1 tsp ground cumin
1 tsp dried oregano
1¼ lb/565 g boneless skinless chicken breasts cut into 1-inch pieces
4 oz/115 g sliced shallots
1 medium sweet red pepper, julienned
1 4-oz/115-g tin chopped green chillies
4 oz/115 g chopped pecans, toasted
shredded lettuce
2 medium tomatoes cut into wedges
1 medium ripe avocado, peeled and sliced
tortillas, warmed (optional)

In a bowl, combine 4 tbs of the oil, lime juice, parsley, garlic, cumin and oregano. Pour half into a large resealable plastic bag; add the chicken. Seal bag and turn to coat; refrigerate for 1 hour or overnight. Cover and refrigerate remaining marinade.

Drain and discard marinade from chicken. In a large frying pan, sauté shallots in remaining oil for 2 minutes. Add chicken; stir-fry for 2–3 minutes or until chicken just begins to brown. Add the red pepper, chillies and reserved marinade; stir-fry for 2 minutes. Stir in pecans.

Place lettuce on individual plates; top with chicken mixture, tomatoes and avocado. Serve with tortillas if desired.

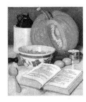 # VEGETABLE DISHES

Stuffed green bell peppers

4 green bell peppers, cored
16 fl oz/450 ml water
7 oz/200 g brown rice
1 lb/455 g lean minced beef
2 oz/55 g chopped onion
½ tsp garlic salt
½ tsp ground black pepper
1 15-oz/425-g tin diced tomatoes
8 oz/225 g shredded cheddar cheese

Parboil the peppers (adding enough water to cover the peppers and bringing them to a boil, then removing from heat). Place in a large baking dish.

Bring water to a boil in a saucepan, add rice. Simmer, covered, for 45 minutes or until rice fluffs with a fork.

Brown minced beef and onion in a frying pan; drain if necessary. Season with garlic salt and pepper. Add rice and tomatoes to the minced beef. Spoon equal portions of the mixture into the peppers, allowing excess mixture to spill into the baking dish.

Sprinkle peppers with shredded cheese and bake in a 350°F/180°C/Gas Mark 4 oven for 30 minutes.

Cranberry rice with caramelized onions

20 fl oz/570 ml chicken broth
3½ oz/100 g uncooked wild rice
3½ oz/100 g uncooked brown rice
3 medium onions cut into wedges
2 tsp brown sugar
3 tbs butter or margarine
5 oz/140 g dried cranberries
½ tsp grated orange peel

In a large saucepan, bring broth to a boil. Add the wild rice. Reduce heat; cover and simmer for 10 minutes. Add the brown rice; cover and simmer for 45–50 minutes or until rice is tender and liquid is absorbed.

In a large frying pan over medium heat, cook the onions and brown sugar in butter until golden brown, stirring frequently. Add the cranberries, orange peel and rice; heat through.

Beans and greens

8 oz/225 g dry Great Northern beans, navy beans, pinto beans, or kidney beans
32 fl oz/900 ml cold water

1 14½-oz/410-g tin reduced-sodium chicken broth
1 bay leaf
1 tsp dried thyme, crushed
¼ tsp ground black pepper
4 slices bacon
1 medium onion, chopped (2 oz/55 g)
1 clove garlic, minced
¼ tsp crushed red pepper (optional)
8 oz/225 g torn mustard greens or spinach
12 oz/340 g chopped tomato (optional)

Rinse beans. In a large saucepan, combine beans and half the water. Bring to boiling; reduce heat and simmer for 2 minutes. Remove from heat. Cover; let stand 1 hour.

Drain and rinse beans. Return beans to the saucepan and add 16 fl oz/450 ml fresh cold water, chicken broth, bay leaf, thyme and black pepper. Bring to boiling; reduce heat. Cover and simmer about 1¼ hours or until the beans are tender, stirring occasionally. (Add more water if needed to prevent sticking or burning.)

Meanwhile, fry the bacon over medium heat until crisp. Drain on paper towels, reserving 1 tbs of dripping in the frying pan. Add onion, garlic, and crushed red pepper, if desired. Cook and stir over medium heat until onion is tender.

Add greens and tomato, if desired, to frying pan. Cover and cook 1 to 2 minutes.

Drain beans, reserving liquid if desired. Discard bay leaf. Return beans to saucepan. Add onion mixture, tossing gently to combine. Season with additional salt and pepper. Spoon into serving bowl. Crumble bacon over top and, if desired, pour reserved liquid over.

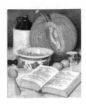 # BREADS AND DESSERTS

Spicy carrot-cake bars

non-stick cooking spray
7½ oz/215 g all-purpose flour
1½ tsp ground cinnamon
¾ tsp ground nutmeg
½ tsp baking powder
¼ tsp ground allspice
4 fl oz/115 ml vegetable oil
7 oz/200 g firmly packed brown sugar
2 eggs
12 oz/340 g shredded carrots
1 8-oz/225-g tin crushed pineapple in juice, drained
1 3-oz/85-g package cream cheese, softened to room temperature
2 oz/55 g sugar
1 tbs all-purpose flour
1 egg
½ tsp lemon juice

Heat oven to 350°F/180°C/Gas Mark 4. Grease a 9 × 13-inch baking pan with nonstick cooking spray. In a medium bowl, combine the flour, cinnamon, nutmeg, baking powder and allspice. Set aside.

In a large bowl, using a wire whisk, beat oil, brown sugar, and eggs until well blended, about 1 minute. Stir in shredded carrots, pineapple, and flour mixture until just blended. Spread batter evenly in pan.

For the topping, in a small bowl, using a wire whisk, beat together cream cheese, sugar and flour until creamy. Add egg and lemon juice; beat well. Drop spoonfuls of cream-cheese filling onto the batter in a random pattern. Using a table knife, cut through the mixture to create a marbled effect.

Bake 25 minutes or until the top is set and the edges pull away from the sides of the pan. Transfer pan to a wire rack and cool completely. Cut into 32 bars.

High-fibre oat bread

1 medium potato, peeled and sliced
water
2 tbs honey
5 oz/140 g wholewheat flour
5 oz/140 g unbleached flour
2½ tsp baking soda
1 tsp cream of tartar
2 oz/55 g rolled oats
2 oz/55 g currants or raisins
cooking spray

Preheat oven to 375°F/190°C/Gas Mark 5. Place the peeled and sliced potato in a small saucepan with water to cover and cook until tender. Drain potato, reserving 6 fl oz/170 ml of the potato water. Mash the potato. Add 4 oz/115 g mashed potato and honey to reserved potato water, stirring well.

Into a medium bowl, sift together the flours, soda, and cream of tartar. Stir in oats and currants.

Make a well in the centre of the dry ingredients and pour in the potato mixture. Stir until a stiff dough forms. Turn out onto a floured board and knead 1 minute with floured hands. Shape into a ball. Place in an 8-inch round cake pan that has been coated with vegetable cooking spray, and flatten slightly. With a sharp knife, make a cross-slash in the top of the loaf.

Bake until the loaf sounds hollow when tapped, 25 to 35 minutes. Serve plain or with fruit butter, jam, honey or a slice of cheese. For best slicing, cool completely before slicing.

Berry Dutch baby

3 large egg whites (reserve yolks for another use)
2 large eggs
5 oz/140 g all-purpose flour
8 fl oz/225 ml non-fat milk
2 tbs granulated sugar
2 tsp vanilla
pinch of salt
1 tbs butter or margarine
12 oz/340 g raspberries or sliced strawberries, or a combination
5 oz/140 g blueberries
¼ tsp ground cinnamon
powdered sugar for garnish

In a blender or food processor, whirl egg whites, eggs, flour, milk, sugar, vanilla, and salt until smooth. Put butter in a 10- to 12-inch non-stick, ovenproof frying pan (preferably with sloping sides) and place in a 425°F/220°C/Gas Mark 7 oven until melted (about 4 minutes). Tip pan to coat evenly. Pour batter into pan and bake until puffed and well browned, about 25 minutes.

Meanwhile, combine berries and cinnamon in a bowl. Spoon berry mixture onto pancake; sprinkle with powdered sugar. Cut into wedges and serve immediately.

Banana-nut muffins

4 eggs, slightly beaten
20 oz/565 g sugar
16 fl oz/450 ml oil

10 oz/285 g mashed ripe bananas (about 3 large)
20 oz/565 g flour
2 tsp baking soda
1½ tsp cinnamon
1 tsp nutmeg
1 tsp ground cloves
1 tsp ground allspice
8 oz/225 g chopped walnuts
5 oz/140 g golden raisins

Topping
2 oz/55 g sugar
½ tsp cinnamon

Combine eggs, sugar, oil and bananas. Mix well. Combine flour, baking soda, cinnamon, nutmeg, cloves and allspice; add to banana mixture along with the walnuts and raisins. Combine just until blended. Divide batter into 24 greased or paper-lined muffin tins. For the topping, combine the sugar and cinnamon and sprinkle over muffins. Bake in preheated 350°F/180°C/Gas Mark 4 oven for 30 minutes.

Carrot-orange bars

5 oz/140 g all-purpose flour
1 tsp baking powder
¼ tsp baking soda
½ tsp ground cinnamon
1 large egg
1 large egg white
7 oz/200 g packed brown sugar
2 tbs canola oil
2 tbs butter or trans fat-free margarine, melted
grated peel and juice of 1 orange
1 tsp vanilla
3 oz/85 g packed grated carrots

2½ oz/70 g raisins
2 oz/55 g dried cranberries or chopped dried apricots
1 oz/30 g chopped walnuts or pecans
cooking spray

Preheat oven to 350°F/180°C/Gas Mark 4. Combine flour, baking powder, baking soda and cinnamon. In a separate bowl, beat egg and egg white until foamy. Beat in sugar, oil, butter, orange peel and juice and vanilla until smooth. Add flour mixture and stir by hand until almost combined. Stir in carrots, fruit and nuts just until blended. Spread batter into 8 × 8-inch pan coated with cooking spray. Bake for 30–35 minutes, until top springs back when lightly touched. Cool in pan on rack.

Oatmeal and wholewheat banana bread

6 oz/170 g mashed ripe bananas (about 2 large)
3 fl oz/90 ml low-fat buttermilk
2 fl oz/60 ml vegetable oil
1 tsp vanilla
2 large eggs, lightly beaten
7½ oz/215 g wholewheat flour
4 oz/115 g light brown sugar
1½ tsp baking powder
¼ tsp baking soda
pinch salt
3 oz/85 g rolled oats
cooking spray

Preheat oven to 350°F/180°C/Gas Mark 4. Combine mashed bananas, buttermilk, vegetable oil, vanilla and eggs in a medium mixing bowl.

In a separate bowl combine flour, brown sugar, baking powder, baking soda, salt and oats. Gradually add banana mixture and stir until moist. Transfer to an 8 × 4-inch bread loaf pan coated with cooking spray.

Bake for 55 minutes or until a wooden testing pick inserted in centre comes out clean. Cool for 15 minutes in pan on a wire rack. Remove from pan and allow to cool completely on wire rack. Slice and serve.

Berry parfait

1 8-oz/225-g container low-fat vanilla yogurt
4 oz/115 g low-fat muesli
5 oz/140 g fresh (or frozen and slightly thawed) blueberries, raspberries or strawberries

In a parfait or tall glass, sprinkle one-third of the muesli, one-third of the yogurt and one-third of the berries. Repeat layers twice. Serves one.

Resources

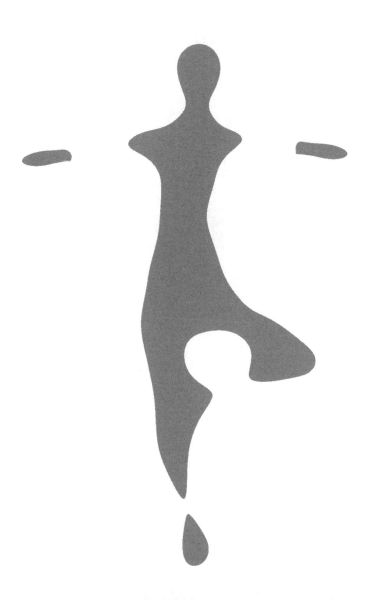

Glossary

Acanthosis nigricans: Velvety and dark skin found on the back of the neck and under the breasts, thought to be associated with obesity and insulin resistance

Acne: Inflammatory disease that affects the sebaceous glands of the skin

Adrenal glands: Gland that releases male hormones (androgens) as well as the stress hormones cortisol and adrenaline

Alopecia: Hair loss

Amenorrhoea: Absence of periods for over three months

Androgen: A group of sex hormones responsible for male sexual characteristics. All female hormones are made from male hormones, and certain amounts are necessary in all women.

Anorexia nervosa: A serious eating disorder whereby the person starves herself

Anovulation: Absence of ovulation

Anti-oestrogen: A substance that mimics or blocks the action of oestrogen

Antioxidants: Vitamins A, C, E and beta-carotene, found in coloured (non-green) fruits and vegetables. Antioxidants prevent the oxidation of cell membranes which can lead to cancer; they are the cancer-fighting soldiers.

Atherosclerosis: Hardening of the arteries due to lipids and plaque formation, associated with hypertension and increased risk of heart disease

Blood sugar: Level of glucose present in the bloodstream, used by the brain and muscles for energy

Bulimia: A serious eating disorder characterized by bingeing then purging through vomiting

Cardiovascular disease: Alteration of the blood vessels of the body, making the individual more prone to decreased muscle function, clot formation and stroke

Cholesterol: Waxy substance found in animal fat. In excess it may contribute to narrowing the artery walls, reducing blood flow.

Clomiphene citrate: Drug most commonly used to induce ovulation. Brand name Clomid.

Corpus luteum: The empty follicle that once held the egg before ovulation

Cortisol: An adrenal hormone involved in stress

Cysts: Masses in ovaries, breasts and elsewhere which are often filled with fluid and are often benign

Diabetes: A condition in which the body either does not use insulin efficiently (Type II diabetes) or does not produce insulin at all (Type I diabetes) resulting in abnormal blood sugar levels

Endocrine: Pertaining to the system of the body that produces hormones

Endocrinologist: A specialist of the endocrine system, the body system that controls all hormonal secretion and function

Endocrinology: The study of the hormone-producing organs, the hormones they produce, their action and interrelationships

Endometriosis: A condition where cells identical to the lining of the uterus (endometrium) are present and growing in a site other than the uterine lining. Associated with chronic inflammation, adhesion formation, progressive pelvic pain and infertility.

Endometrial hyperplasia: Overgrowth of the uterine lining (endometrium) usually due to the influence of prolonged oestrogen exposure

Endometrium: Lining of the uterus

Enzyme: A protein that facilitates biochemical reactions

Essential fatty acids: Crucial nutrients for cells, which also regulate hormone production

Fibre: Part of a plant that cannot be digested, which can lower cholesterol levels or improve regularity; also causes a slower rise in glucose levels, which lowers the body's insulin requirements

Fibroid: A benign fibrous tumour of the uterine muscle

Follicle: A small fluid-filled sac in the ovary that contains an egg. The follicle ruptures and releases an egg at ovulation.

Follicle-stimulating hormone (FSH): A hormone produced by the pituitary gland that promotes the ovarian follicle development

Free radical: An electron-poor substance that can bind to lipids and other substances, triggering an immune response, destruction or ageing

Gene: Basic unit of heredity; bits of DNA working together to achieve a single function

Gestational diabetes: The development of diabetes during pregnancy

Glucose: Food is digested and converted to glucose, which is also called blood sugar and is a source of energy that circulates in the bloodstream

Glucose tolerance test (GTT): A test to exclude altered carbohydrate metabolism and diabetes. A sweetened drink with a known amount of glucose is given and blood tests for glucose levels are repeated at intervals.

Glycaemic Index: The measure of how a standard number of calories from a given food affects blood sugar. The faster a food is digested and the more calories it contains, the more blood sugar levels will spike.

HDL: High-density lipoproteins, known as 'good' cholesterol

High blood pressure: Condition in which the heart pumps blood through the circulatory system at a pressure greater than normal. Normal blood pressure is usually below 140/90. Also called hypertension.

Hirsutism: An increase in the amount and/or coarseness of hair distributed in the male pattern in a female

Hormone: A substance made in small quantities by an (endocrine)

organ which is secreted into the blood and has its effects on distant and specific cells, tissues or organs

Hyperandrogenism: Condition in which a woman has high levels of male sex hormones (androgens)

Hyperglycaemia: Elevated blood sugar levels

Hyperinsulinaemia: Elevated insulin levels

Hyperplasia: Overgrowth of cells

Hypertension: Elevated blood pressure where the systolic (top number) is greater than 140 and the diastolic (bottom number) is greater than 90

Hypoglycaemia: Low levels of blood sugar

Hypothalamus: Part of the brain responsible for maintaining body temperature, sleep, hunger and reproduction

Hypothyroidism: Condition characterized by an underactive thyroid

Infertility: The inability to conceive after a year of unprotected intercourse, or to carry a pregnancy to term

Insulin: A hormone produced by the pancreas that regulates the energy use of the body. Insulin converts glucose from the bloodstream into glycogen, which is stored in muscle tissue and the liver

Insulin resistance: A condition where the body steadily becomes less responsive to the actions of insulin. Related to diabetes.

Insulin sensitizers: Group of medications originally used to treat diabetes but now sometimes used to alleviate many PCOS-related symptoms by helping to correct insulin resistance

LDL: Low-density lipoproteins, known as 'bad' cholesterol

Laparoscopy: A surgical procedure usually performed in an outpatient setting in which a small telescope is inserted through an abdominal incision to examine the ovaries, uterus and fallopian tubes

Luteinizing hormone (LH): Hormone produced and released by the pituitary gland. In a woman it's responsible for ovulation and the maintenance of the corpus luteum

Menopause: When menstruation has stopped for at least one year — usually around age 45 to 50. Once this occurs, a woman is no longer able to get pregnant

Menses: Approximately monthly discharge of the unfertilized egg and the uterine lining as blood flows through the vagina

Menstruation: Monthly cycle of hormone production and ovarian activities that prepares the body for pregnancy. If pregnancy does not occur, the uterine lining is shed, causing menses

Metabolic syndrome – Syndrome X: Disorder characterized by insulin resistance, hypertension and abnormal cholesterol

Obesity: An excessive storage of body fat: a weight more than 20 per cent above average

Oestrogen: The major female reproductive hormone

Omega-3 fatty acids: Naturally present in fish that swim in cold waters; crucial for brain tissue; are all polyunsaturated, and not only lower cholesterol levels but are said to protect against heart disease

Osteoporosis: The most common bone disease, characterized by reduced bone mineral density and deterioration of the internal structural support within the bones, leading to increased bone fragility and fracture

Ovaries: The female sex glands which produce eggs and secrete the hormones oestrogen and progesterone

Ovulation: The releasing of a mature egg (ovum) from a follicle every month

Pituitary gland: An organ located at the base of the brain that produces hormones which regulate the menstrual cycle

Progesterone: A hormone produced by the corpus luteum of the ovary after ovulation has occurred that prepares the uterus for a pregnancy

Progestin: A synthetic agent that mimics the action of progesterone

Proteins: Compounds that contain amino acids. Found in all living matter, proteins are essential for the growth and repair of animal tissue.

Saturated fat: A fat solid at room temperature (from animal sources) that stimulates the body to produce LDL, or bad cholesterol

Sex hormone binding globulin (SHBG): A blood test used as a marker for PCOS. Low levels are an indication of insulin resistance. Age, weight, diet and hormone levels all affect the concentration of SHBG

Soluble fibre: Fibre that is water soluble or dissolves in water, forms a gel in the body that traps fats and lowers cholesterol

Stroke: Occurs when a blood clot travels to the brain and stops the flow of blood and oxygen carried to the nerve cells in that area, at which point cells may die or vital body functions, controlled by the brain, may be temporarily or permanently damaged

Syndrome: A specific disorder characterized by a unified and identified group of signs and symptoms

Syndrome X: See Metabolic syndrome

Testosterone: The principal male sex hormone

Thyroid gland: An endocrine gland in the front and the base of the neck that regulates general body metabolism, including hormone balance in the body

Transfatty acids (hydrogenated oils): Harmful, man-made fats that not only raise the level of bad cholesterol (LDL) in the bloodstream but lower the amount of good cholesterol (HDL) that's already there; produced through the process of hydrogenation

Triglycerides: A combination of saturated, monounsaturated and polyunsaturated fatty acids and glycerol

Ultrasound: Imaging technique where sound waves are passed through a hand-held transducer so tissues can be examined. The technique can be placed in the vagina to enable the best visualization of the ovaries and the uterus, but it can also be performed on the abdomen (though the bladder must be very full to allow the best image)

Unsaturated fat: Known as good fat because it doesn't cause the body to produce bad cholesterol and it increases the level of good cholesterol, partially solid or liquid at room temperature

Uterus: A pear-shaped reproductive organ of the female that nurtures the developing baby until birth

Waist—hip ratio: Distance around the mid-portion, greatest diameter of the hip divided by the waist measurement. Often used to define type of obesity and specific disease risks

Withdrawal bleeding: Menses produced by giving medication, such as Provera, to induce a period

Useful Contacts

If you want to find out more about PCOS in general or hook up with other women with PCOS or find out more about the health risks associated with PCOS, these are some of the most relevant contacts and websites. Remember, the beauty of websites is that they are international so you can get some great help and information from any of the websites listed here, not just from organizations based in your country. If you do write to an organization, always send a stamped addressed envelope, as many of these are charities run by volunteers.

In addition to your doctor's advice, a PCOS support group should be your first port of call. Groups like Verity in the UK or PCOS Support in the US can help put you in touch with a support group in your area and also give you the advice, support and information you need to make informed choices about PCOS and your health and well-being.

UK

PCOS
Verity
Graystone Street
28 Charles Square
London N1 6HT
www.verity-pcos.org.uk

Verity has loads of information and
advice for women with PCOS, details
of events and other items of news.

CANCER
Cancer Research UK
PO Box 123
Lincoln's Inn Fields
London WC2A 3PX
Te: 020 7242 0200

COMPLEMENTARY THERAPIES
British Complementary Medicine Association
St Charles Hospital
Exmoor Street
London W10 6DZ
Tel: 020 8964 1205

Council for Complementary and Alternative Medicine
179 Gloucester Place
London NW1 6DX
Tel: 020 7724 9103

COUNSELLING/DEPRESSION
The Samaritans
24-hour helpline: 0845 790 9090

British Association for Counselling
1 Regent Place
Rugby
Warwickshire CV21 2PJ

Depression Alliance
35 Westminster Bridge Road
London SE1 7JB
Tel: 020 7633 0557

MIND – Mental Health Charity
15–19 Broadway
London E15 4BQ
Tel: 0845 766 0163

DIABETES
Diabetes UK
10 Parkway
London NW1 7AA
Tel: 020 7424 1000

DIET AND NUTRITION
British Dietetic Association
5th Floor, Charles House
148–149 Great Charles Street
Birmingham B3 3HT
Tel: 0121 200 8080

British Nutrition Foundation
High Holborn House
52 High Holborn
London WC1V 6RQ
Tel: 020 7404 6504

Institute for Optimum Nutrition
Blades Court
Deodar Road
London SW15 2NU
Tel: 020 8877 9993

Vegetarian Society
Parkdale
Denham Road
Altrincham
Cheshire WA14 4QS
Tel: 0161 928 0793

Vegan Society
Donald Watson House
7 Battle Road
St Leonard's on Sea
East Sussex TN3 7AA
Tel: 01424 427 393

EATING DISORDERS
Eating Disorders Association
103 Prince of Wales Road
Norfolk NR1 1DW
Tel: 0845 634 1414

Overeaters Anonymous
Tel: 01273 624 712
Nationwide local groups throughout
the UK

HEART HEALTH
British Cardiac Society
9 Fitzroy Square
London W1P 5AH
Tel: 020 7383 3887

British Heart Foundation
14 Fitzhardinge Street
London W1H 4DH
Tel: 020 7388 0903

British Hypertension Society Information
Service
Blood Pressure Unit
Department of Medicine
St George's Hospital Medical School
Cranmer Terrace
London SW17 ORE
Tel: 020 725 3412

SUPPLEMENTS
Biocare Nutritional Supplements
Tel: 0121 433 3727

The Herbalists' Center
Tel: 0207 935 0405

The Nutri Centre
Tel: 020 7436 5122

Viridian Supplements
Tel: 01327 878050

Nutrition Mission
Tel: 01725 514222

Solgar Vitamins
Tel: 01442 890355

Lambert Healthcare
Tel: 01892 552120

Specialist Herbal Supplies
Tel: 01273 202401

Higher Nature Ltd
Tel: 01435 882880

Health Plus Ltd
Tel: 01323 737374

WEIGHT LOSS
Lighten Up
46 Staines Road
Twickenham TW2 5AH
Tel: 0845 603 3456

Vitaline Weight Control Ltd
144 Ashton Road
Manchester M34 3HR
Tel: 0161 292 4918

WOMEN'S HEALTH
Women's Health
52 Featherstone Street
London EC1Y 8RT
Tel: 020 7251 6580

Smoking Quitline
NHS helpline
Tel: 0800 1690169

US

PCOS
Polycystic Ovarian Syndrome Association Inc., PCOSA
PO Box 80517
Portland, OR 97280
www.pcosupport.org

PCOSA is the US-based self-help group to which Verity in the UK is affiliated. A treasure trove of information, advice, help and support.

CANCER
American Cancer Society
1955 Clifton Road
Atlanta, GA 30329
Tel: 1-800-ACS 2345

National Cancer Institute
Building 41, Room 10A24
9000 Rockville Pike
Bethesda, MD 20892
Tel: 800-4-CANCER

COMPLEMENTARY/ ALTERNATIVE THERAPIES
National Clearing House for Complementary and Alternative Medicine
PO Box 8218
Silver Spring, MD 20907-8218
Tel: 1-888-664-6226

COUNSELLING/DEPRESSION
Concerned Counselling
Telephone counselling service toll-free within the US: 1-888-415-8255

National Foundation for Depressive Illness
PO Box 2257
New York, NY 10016
Tel: 212 268 4260

DIABETES
National Diabetes Information Clearing House (NDIC)
1 Information Way
Bethesda, MD 20892–3560
Tel: 301 654 3810

American Diabetes Association
1701 North Beauregard Street
Alexandria, VA 22311

DIET AND NUTRITION
The American Dietetic Association
216 West Jackson Boulevard
Chicago, IL 60606 6995
Tel: 312 899 0040

Food and Nutrition Information Center
National Agriculture Library
10301 Baltimore Avenue
Room 304
Beltsville, MD 20705-2351
Tel: 301 504 5719

North American Vegetarian Society
PO Box 72Q
Dolgeville, NY 13329
Tel: 518-568-7970

American Vegan Society
56 Dinshah Lane
PO Box 369
Malaga, NJ 08328
Tel: 856-694-2887

EATING DISORDERS
American Anorexia/Bulimia Association
418E 76th Street
New York, NY 10021
Tel: 212 734 1114

HEART DISEASE
The American Heart Association
7272 Greenville Avenue
Dallas, TX 75231
Tel: 214 762 6300
(also provides information about
hypertension)

SUPPLEMENTS
Bleser Herbs
Tel: 800 489 4372

Herbal Magic Inc.
Tel: 415 488 9488

Herbal Pharmacy
Tel: 541 846 6262

May Way Trading
Tel: 510 208 3113

Metagenics
Tel: 800 692 9400

Nature's Apothecary
Tel: 303 581 0288

Uni Key Health Systems
Tel: 800 888 4353

*International Academy of Compounding
Pharmacists*
Tel: 713 933 8400

Will help you locate a local pharmacy
that specializes in natural prescriptions

WOMEN'S HEALTH
*National Women's Health Resource Center
(NWHRC)*
120 Albany Street
Suite 820
New Brunswick, NJ 08901
Tel: 877 986 9742

National clearing-house for information, internet links and resources about
women's health

AUSTRALIA

*POSAA – Polycystic Ovary Syndrome
Association of Australia*
PO Box E140
Emerton
NSW 2770
Tel: 612 4733 4342
www.posaa.asn.au

Diabetes Australia
AVA House
5/7 Phipps Place
Deakin
ACT 2600
Tel: 616 285 3277

Women's Health Statewide
64 Pennington Terrace
Nth Adelaide SA 5006
Tel: 08 8267 5366

WEBSITES

PCOS

www.verity-pcos.org.uk

www.pcosupport.org – US PCOS
support group website affiliated to
Verity in the UK

www.posaa.asn.au – Australian support
group website

www.pcosupport.org/pcoteen/about.ht
ml – PCOTeen is a division of
PCOSA for women in their teens
with PCOS

www.pcos.net – 'Helping women with
PCOS' is the motto of this friendly
US website which includes info on
low-carb diets and ongoing research

www.pcos-equality.org.uk – Campaign
group set up by women to fight the
'postcode lottery' that exists in the
UK when applying for laser treatment for excess hair

www.soulcysters.com – US-based e-
group for women with PCOS to
meet and exchange information

www.pcolist.org/mailman/listinfo/
thincysters – US based e-group for
cysters within the normal weight
range

Complementary and alternative medicine

www.bcma.co.uk

http: //nccam.nih.gov

www.internethealthlibrary.com

www.bloom.com.au

Glycaemic Index

www.glycemicindex.com

Information on the glycaemic index of
foods, latest GI data, books and
testing services

www.gidiet.com

A detailed guide to the GI diet, which
also offers you the opportunity to
submit any of your experiences with
the GI diet and any tips, suggestions
or recipes

Diabetes

www.diabetes.org

www.diabetes.org.uk

www.mendosa.com/org.htm

Amazing website which links you to
every other useful website on
diabetes/insulin resistance

Cancer

www.cancer.org
www.cancerresearchuk.org
www.nci.nih.gov

Heart health/hypertension

www.bcs.com
www.bhf.org.uk
www.hyp.ac.uk/bhsinfo
www.familyheart.org
www.americanheart.org

Nutrition

www.eatright.org

www.thefooddoctor.co.uk
www.naturopathic.org
www.patrickholford.com

Thyroid

www.thyroiduk.org
www.thyroid.com

Women's health

www.obgyn.net
www.nlm.nih.gov
www.healthywoman.org
www.whas.com.au

Further Reading

PCOS

Colette Harris and Dr Adam Carey: *PCOS: A Woman's Guide to Dealing with Polycystic Ovary Syndrome* (Thorsons)
Colette Harris and Theresa Cheung: *The PCOS Diet Book* (Thorsons)
Colette Harris and Theresa Cheung: *PCOS and Your Fertility* (Hay House)
Dr Samuel Thatcher: *PCOS: The Hidden Epidemic* (Perspectives Press)

BODY IMAGE

Thomas Cash: *Body Image Workshop* (New Harbinger)
Barbara Harris and Angela Hynes: *Shape Your Life: Four Weeks to a Better Body and a Better Life* (Hay House)
Marcia Hutchinson: *200 Ways to Love the Body You Have* (Crossing)

CANCER

Kerry McGlinn and Pamela Haylock: *Women's Cancers: How to Prevent them, How to Treat Them, How to Beat Them* (Hunter House)

COMPLEMENTARY/ALTERNATIVE/HERBAL MEDICINE

Kitty Campion: *Holistic Women's Herbal* (Bloomsbury)
Susan Clarke: *What Really Works: The Insiders Guide to Natural Medicine* (Bantam)

Amanda Crawford: *Herbal Remedies for Women* (Prima)
Jennifer Harper: *Nine Ways to Body Wisdom* (Thorsons)
Tori Hudson: *Women's Encyclopedia of Natural Medicine* (McGraw Hill)

DIET/NUTRITION

Jenny Bowden: *Living the Low Carb Life — from Atkins to the Zone — Choosing the Diet that's Right for You* (Sterling)
Jean Carper: *Food — Your Miracle Medicine* (Simon and Schuster)
June Clarke: *Body Foods for Women* (Orion)
Cheryl Hart and Mary Kay Grossman: *The Insulin Resistance Diet* (Contemporary Books)
Gillian Mckeith: *You Are What You Eat* (Michael Joseph)
Maryon Stewart: *Beat Sugar Cravings: The Revolutionary Four-week Diet* (Vermilion)

DETOX

Ann Louise Gittleman: *The Living Beauty Detox Programme* (Harper San Francisco)
Suzannah Oliver: *The Detox Manual* (Pocket Books)
Amanda Ursell: *Cleanse Your System* (Thorsons)

DIABETES

Rudy Bilous: *Understanding Diabetes* (British Medical Association)
Vern Cherewatenko and Paul Perry: *The Diabetes Cure* (Thorsons)
Kaye Foster-Powell: *The Glucose Revolution* (Hodder Mobius)
Milton Hammerly: *Diabetes — How to Combine the Best of Traditional and Alternative Therapies* (Adams Media)

Annette Maggi and Jackie Boucher: *What You Can Do to Prevent Diabetes* (Wiley)

Prevention: Outsmart Diabetes (St Martin's Paperbacks)

EATING DISORDERS

Diana Cassel: *Food for Thought – Sourcebook for Obesity and Eating Disorders* (Facts on File)

Carolyn Costin: *The Eating Disorder Sourcebook* (McGraw Hill)

Jane Hirshmann and Carol Munter: *When Women Stop Hating Their Bodies – Freeing Yourself from Food and Weight Obsession* (Ballantine)

Marilyn Migliore and Philip Ross: *The Hunger Within – A Twelve Week Self Guided Journey from Compulsive Eating to Recovery* (Doubleday)

Richard Oakes-Ash: *Good Girls Do Swallow* (Mainstream Publishing)

ENDOMETRIOSIS

Dian Shepperson Mills and Michael Vernon: *Endometriosis – A Key to Healing through Nutrition* (Thorsons)

FATIGUE

Erica White: *The Beat Fatigue Handbook* (Thorsons)

FITNESS

Rosemary Conley Fitness Videos, BBC Worldwide and video collection, inc VHS

Sally Gunnel: *Be Your Best* (Thorsons)

Howard Kent: *The Complete Illustrated Guide to Yoga* (Element)

FOOD AND MOOD

Amanda Geary: *The Food and Mood Handbook* (Thorsons)
Elizabeth Somer: *Food and Mood* (Owl Books)

GIVING UP SMOKING

Allen Carr's Easy Way to Stop Smoking (Penguin)
Susannah Hayward: *Breathe Easy — The Friendly Stop Smoking Guide for Women* (Penguin)

GLYCAEMIC INDEX

Dr Stephen Colagiuri: *The Glucose Revolution* (Hodder and Stoughton)
Rick Gallop: *The GI Diet* (Virgin)
Anthony Leeds: *The GI Factor* (Hodder and Stoughton)
Jeanie Brand Miller and Thomas Wolever: *The New Glucose Revolution — The Authoritative Guide to the Glycemic Index — The Dietary Solution for Lifelong Health* (Marlowe and Company)
Nigel Denby: *The GL Diet: Diet Freedom* (Blake Publishing)

HEART HEALTH/HYPERTENSION

Chris Davidson: *Understanding Coronary Heart Disease* (British Medical Association)
Louise Hay: *Heart Thoughts — Treasury of Inner Wisdom* (Hay House)
Prevention: Outsmart High Blood Pressure (St Martin's Paperbacks)
Sara Rosenthal: *50 Ways Women can Prevent Heart Disease* (Lowell House)
Stephen Sinatra: *Heart Sense for Women — Your Plan for Natural Prevention and Treatment* (Lifeline Press)

HORMONES

Theresa Cheung: *Androgen Disorders in Women* (Hunter House)
Gale Maleskey and Marry Kittel: *The Hormone Connection* (Rodale Press)
Kate Neil and Patrick Holford: *Balancing Hormones Naturally* (Piatkus)
Geoffrey Redmond: *The Good News about Women's Hormones* (Warner)

ORGANIC LIVING

Lynda Brown: *Organic Living – Simple Strategies for a Better Life*
Maurice Hansen and Jill Marsden: *E is for Additives* (Thorsons)
Karen Sullivan: *Organic Living in 10 Simple Lesson* (Barnes Ed)

STRESS/SELF-ESTEEM/LIFE SKILLS

David Burns: *10 Days to Great Self-esteem* (Vermilion)
Louise Hay: *Affirmations for Self-Esteem* (Hay House)
Louise Hay: *The Power is Within You* (Hay House)
Louise Hay: *Heal Your Life* (Hay House)
Robert Holden: *Stressbusters* (Thorsons)
Cathy Hopkins: *101 Shortcuts to Relaxation* (Bloomsbury)
Phil McGraw: *Life Strategies* (Free Press)
Matthew McKay: *Self-Esteem Companion* (New Harbinger)
Paul McKenna: *Change Your life in Seven Days* (Bantam)
Kenneth Matheny: *Write Your Own Prescription for Stress* (New Harbinger)
Paul Wilson: *The Little Book of Calm* (Penguin)

SUPPLEMENTS

James and Phyliss Balch: *Prescription for Nutritional Healing* (Avery)
Patrick Holford: *The Optimum Nutrition Bible* (Piatkus)

Linda Lazarides: *the Nutritional Health Bible* (Thorsons)
Earl Mindel's Supplement Bible (Thorsons)

SYNDROME X/METABOLIC DISORDER

Jack Challem: *Syndrome X: Complete Nutritional Programme for Insulin Resistance* (John Wiley)
Cheryl Hart: *The Insulin Resistance Diet* (McGraw Hill)
Anthony Haynes: *The Insulin Factor* (Thorsons)

THYROID

Martin Budd: *Why Am I so Tired? Is Your Thyroid Making You Ill* (Thorsons)

WEIGHT LOSS

Pete Cohen and Judith Verity: *Lighten Up* (Century)
Phil McGraw: *The Ultimate Weight Solution* (Free Press)
Barry Sears: *The Zone – A Dietary Road Map to Lose Weight Permanently* (Harper Collins)

WELL WOMAN

Joan Borysenko: *A Woman's Book of Life* (Riverhead Books)
Marilyn Glenville: *The Natural Health Handbook for Women* (Piatkus)
Louise Hay: *Heal Your Body* (Hay House)
Christiane Northrup: *Women's Bodies, Women's Wisdom* (Bantam)

General Index

Please note that cancers are filed under their respective sites, e.g. breast cancer is filed under b. Tables are indicated by *italic* page numbers and main references are in **bold**. A separate index is provided for the recipes.

Index of Recipes

The index enables quick location of the recipies in Part Four. For all other items, please refer to the General Index.

Notes

Notes

We hope you enjoyed this Hay House book.
If you would like to receive a free catalogue featuring additional
Hay House books and products, or if you would like information
about the Hay Foundation, please contact:

Hay House UK Ltd

Unit 62, Canalot Studios • 222 Kensal Rd • London W10 5BN
Tel: (44) 20-8962-1230; Fax: (44) 20-8962-1239
www.hayhouse.co.uk

Published and distributed in the United States of America by:
Hay House, Inc. • P.O. Box 5100 • Carlsbad, CA 92018-5100
Tel: (1) 760-431-7695 or (800) 654-5126; Fax: (1) 760-431-6948 or (800) 650-5115
www.hayhouse.com

Published and distributed in Australia by:
Hay House Australia Ltd • 18/36 Ralph St • Alexandria NSW 2015
Phone: (61) 2-9669-4299 • Fax: (61) 2-9669-4144
www.hayhouse.com.au

Published and distributed in the Republic of South Africa by:
Hay House SA (Pty) Ltd • PO Box 990 • Witkoppen 2068
Phone/Fax: (27) 11-706-6612 • orders@psdprom.co.za

Distributed in Canada by:
Raincoast • 9050 Shaughnessy St • Vancouver, BC V6P 6E5
Phone: (1) 604 323 7100 • Fax: (1) 604 323 2600

Sign up via the Hay House UK website to receive the Hay House
online newsletter and stay informed about what's going on with
your favourite authors. You'll receive bimonthly announcements
about discounts and offers, special events, product highlights,
free excerpts, giveaways, and more!
www.hayhouse.co.uk